The Ultimate Women's Fat Loss Guide

by Eric Bonilla

All Rights Reserved

About the Author

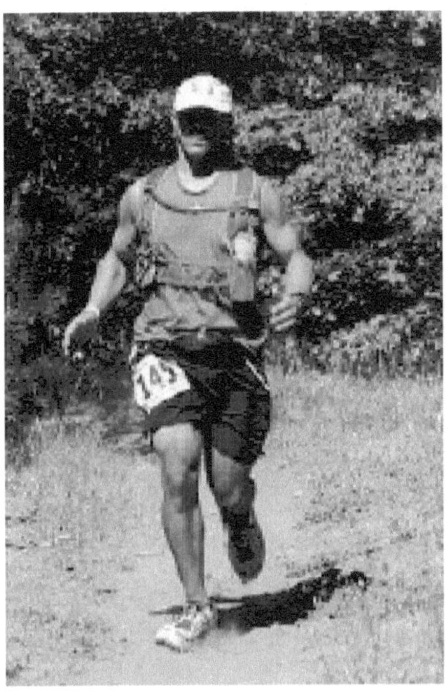

For the last 20 years, Eric Bonilla has been involved in helping women reach their weight loss goals through scientifically-based, proven programs. He has spent hundreds of hours training women and has learned what works and what doesn't work.

This book is the result of 20 years of "In the trenches" work. In this book, Eric has collected a blueprint to your fitness success, which has been proven by hundreds and hundreds of success stories from his gym. Get ready to transform your life!

Table of Contents

Introduction

The Ultimate Women's Fat Loss Guide consists of the best fat-burning, muscle-building exercises and routines that women at my gym perform every day. The Ultimate Women's Fat Loss system also includes a nutritional program with sample meals and fat loss strategies that women of all ages and fitness levels have used to achieve amazing results. Literally thousands of exercises and fat loss programs have come and gone in the fitness arena. Needless to say, the wheel has been invented; nevertheless, we are inundated with books, diets, exercise equipment, and DVDs, mostly from the endless late night infomercials. The very thought of sorting through the madness to find what works and what to throw away can be a daunting task, to say the least. We are left confused and frustrated over wondering which path to travel to attain our fat loss goals.

Finally, there is light at the end of the tunnel. For many years, The Ultimate Fat loss system has brought incredible results for women at my facility, Tried & True. The women at my gym love that they perform the same exercises that athletes perform—of course, at different intensity levels—nevertheless, the exercises are the same and women of all ages gain confidence, self-esteem, and strength from knowing they are capable of conquering The Ultimate Women's Fat Loss System.

The Ultimate Women's Fat Loss program consists of multi-joint movements that work multiple muscles, build more muscle, burn more calories, and, more importantly, burn more fat on your body. These exercises are not only great because they activate a lot of muscle and burn a huge amount of fat, but they make you better at whatever you need to accomplish in life. For example, a task that was once hard to manage can now be completed with less effort and with energy to spare.

Whether it's carrying the groceries, playing with the grandchildren, or driving a golf ball a couple hundred yards, The Ultimate Fat Loss System for Women will improve every aspect of your life.

Training Basics

Dumbell Training

Dumbbell training is a versatile form of training that allows the body to work unilaterally, where each side of the body works on its own, to ensure that the stronger side doesn't take over the weaker side. This is an important benefit, especially if you have a dominant side of your body. Dumbbell training could be just what the doctor ordered to "clean up" imbalances you've accumulated from years of using your dominant side and neglecting your weaker side. Dumbbell training also strengthens and stabilizes muscles that usually aren't working adequately with other forms of training. In addition, because of the unilateral component, balance is improved as a result of dumbbells. Potentially, dumbbell training has many more movements than other forms of training, which are very important in everyday life.

The Ultimate Women's Fat Loss System focuses on training movements instead of a "bodybuilding" approach to training, where muscles are isolated. A "movements" based approach to training kills not only kills two birds with one stone, it kills multitudes (don't worry, birds are not harmed in the analogy). Seriously, multiple planes, including the transverse plane (splits the upper and lower body in two), the sagital plane (imaginary line that divides the body into left and right halves), and the frontal plane (divides body into front and back halves) are worked. A "movements over muscles" training strategy also prevents injuries because inherent in the training is balance, stabilization, and coordination. In addition, dumbbell training prepares muscles by training the nervous system to move the body more efficiently and with less injury.

Barbell Training

After reading the dumbbell section, please don't throw away all of your barbells. On the contrary, barbell training has been around for a thousand years and will be around for another thousand years. All of the great strong men and women of yesteryear have built their mind-boggling strength and super-human conditioning by using barbells. In fact, I believe that barbells are a requirement for any resistance training program and are used in this book. Exercises such as the barbell deadlift, the barbell squat, and the barbell bench press are needed when weights are too heavy to load the body efficiently, and when using a dumbbell wouldn't be a practical choice. Barbells allow you to focus on the load instead of worrying about balancing and stabilizing to the same extent that you would with dumbbells. A balance and coordination challenge exists with barbell training but not to the same extent as with dumbbells.

Developing Overall Fitness

The Ultimate Women's Fat Loss System will not only make you incredibly conditioned, you'll also notice that your strength levels increase dramatically. You will no longer have to worry about asking someone to help you move or lift something in case of emergency, as the added strength will be there for you to utilize. Although many benefits exist with The Ultimate Women's Fat Loss System, its main focus is fat loss. This program is designed to get you in the best possible shape in the shortest length of time.

The Ultimate Women's Fat Loss System is not meant to be a sports performance program, although if you are playing a sport, it will undoubtedly improve your performance. It is a conditioning, fat-burning program to get you in the best shape of your life.

In my gym, all clients are trained to be more efficient at whatever they do. If they are athletes, they become better athletes. General fitness and weekend warriors become better prepared for whatever life might throw at them. It's important to have that reserve of strength and power to get yourself out of a tough situation in life or a last-second play on the field. Other benefits of The Ultimate Women's Fat Loss system are improved flexibility and mobility. You'll find yourself moving more efficiently and with greater range of motion because your body is more flexible. You will need less effort to do the same tasks you did before because your muscles, working as a unit in the gym, will therefore work as a unit outside the gym. Think of the energy that you waste when normal everyday tasks need to be completed and you have flexibility and mobility issues.

Cardio Only?

Beware of becoming a smaller version of what you were. Yes, it's a scary thought, but it will happen. Many diet and training programs have you believe that diet and steady-state cardio will help you get the body you desire. There is no doubt that if you follow a calorie-reducing program, you will lose weight, but at what expense? You will pay dearly with muscle loss, which is the opposite of your goals. Muscle is metabolically active tissue; it speeds up your metabolism, making it possible to burn calories even while you're sleeping. At the very least, we want muscle retention. The best case scenario is one in which we gain muscle, increase metabolism, tone, shed fat and inches, while gaining tons of energy.

Strength Training: The Magic Bullet

We're all looking for the magic bullet that will bring us guaranteed results. Well, in the case of fat loss, strength training is your magic bullet. Tried and true, lifting weights works. Strength training puts muscle on your body, and muscle, a valuable commodity, brings numerous benefits to the person who will put forth the effort and focus to adhere to a strength training program. I often tell my clients that if strength training were easy, everyone would look like Greek goddesses. It's not easy. Strength training requires consistent work, but it can be done. Just remind yourself of all the benefits, such as shedding inches, speeding metabolism, toning and tightening your body, increasing energy levels, and building strength, endurance, power, mobility, and flexibility. The benefits are valuable and far too numerous to pass up. Strength training must be a part of your fat loss program and your life.

Long Slow Distance or L.S.D.

Yes, L.S.D. brings thoughts of a different subject matter altogether. Actually, L.S.D. stands for 'long slow distance,' but like the substance L.S.D., it should be outlawed for the harm it does to your fitness goals. L.S.D. trains the body to become more efficient at fat loss. At a glance, this might seem beneficial, but in actuality, your muscles are shrinking to become more efficient at going long distances. In essence, you are creating a smaller fat burning machine, which allows your body to store more fat because there's less machinery around to burn it. Weight training builds muscle instead of burns muscle, as an adaptation to higher intensity levels. What type of body looks the best, a toned sprinter's body or a marathoner's body? I would rather have the sprinter's body. It's a healthier body and more efficient at burning fat.

Isolationist Training

I didn't coin the term. The late MellSiff used this term to describe exercises that are meant for rehab but are applied to sports training. Isolationist training is training your body one body part at a time (i.e., leg extensions) instead of through movements that work multiple muscles at the same time (i.e., standing shoulder press, power cleans, etc.). Isolationist training is a horrible choice for a fat loss program (sorry, but it's the truth). With only one body part being worked at a time, the caloric expenditure is miniscule compared with doing a clean and jerk or a squat. Moreover, the body is designed to work in unison or as a system of body parts to fulfill movement obligations.

When this intricate system called the human body is programmed to work in different and unproductive ways, the machinery malfunctions and causes problems for the owner. Why would we train the body in a manner that is opposite to how the body functions? I believe that the majority of the injuries witnessed in professional sports are because athletes still train using bodybuilding routines for bodybuilders. That's fine, but for an athlete whose body parts must work in unison, there is no excuse for, or need for, isolationist training. To me, an athlete who trains in a manner completely not in line with his or her performance on the playing field is unbelievable.

Take, for example, sitting in weight machines regardless of your athletic ability, whether it's at the general fitness level or the elite athlete level. Machines groove the range of motion; therefore, they do not create a need for balance or coordination. In addition, the body does not get the benefit of proprioception. For example, leg extensions only work the quadriceps and work one joint—the knee. Squats, on the other hand, bring into play many different muscles and involve three joints: ankle, knee, and hips. Machines serve to rewire the nervous system, like putting a bad program into your computer and deleting the good program that you developed with free weights. Moreover, the design of such machines change posture and body positioning, leading to excessive loading of a joint, which may lead to serious injury where safety was the goal in mind. The bottom line is that machines are made to isolate muscles, not movements. Free weights train movements and muscles, and burn more calories at the same time.

Interval and Circuit Training

Interval training combines high intensity training with lower intensity training. This combination makes training harder possible because the lower intensity work allows the body to recover, ensuring that form and technique do not suffer because of fatigue. The high intensity intervals can be made more difficult and longer, while the rest periods can be shortened. These types of adjustments can continue to be made, with only your imagination to hold you back. Circuit training is set up where one moves from one exercise to the next, with 10 to 15 seconds between exercises. Many different combinations are possible for your circuits. You can follow the order of the exercises provided in this e-book or you can modify them. You are only limited by your imagination. Later on in the e-book, we will go into detail about specific programs.

The following is an example of a Cardio Interval workout utilizing a treadmill. You can also perform the workout outside. Keep track of your intensity levels using the Rate of Perceived Exertion (RPE). The Rate of Perceived Exertion helps you determine your intensity levels. Here are the 10 intensity levels that correspond to different levels of RPE.

1. Sitting down doing nothing
2. Able to continue pace for an extended period

3. Still easy but getting more difficult
4. Starting to sweat but can talk easily
5. Sweating a bit more but still talking easily
6. Can talk, but slightly breathless
7. Sweating big time. Intense pace
8. Can't talk. Pace can be held a short length of time
9. All-out sprint
10. Forget it. Not Happening

This Cardio Interval workout provided is an example. Gauge your level of fitness and perform the workout at the intensity level that you are able to manage.

Duration	Description	RPE
5 Minutes	**Warm up. Start with fast walk or light jog.**	3-4
2 Minutes	**Increase body temperature. Prepare body for higher intensity.**	5
2 Minutes	**Increase pace of jog. First minute, slight increase from jog; slightly faster second minute.**	6-7
2 Minutes	**Continue pace first minute; slightly slower second minute.**	7-6
1 Minute	**Increase speed to sprint.**	8
2 Minutes	**Decrease speed to initial pace.**	5
2 Minutes	**First minute, slight increase from jog; slightly faster second minute.**	6-7

Duration	Description	RPE
2 Minutes	**Continue pace first minute; slightly**	7-6
1 Minute	**slower second minute.**	
	Increase speed to sprint; slightly	8-9
2 Minutes	**faster last thirty seconds.**	
5 Minutes	**Decrease speed to initial pace.**	5
	Cool down: walk at warm-up pace.	3-4
	Total workout time: 26 minutes.	

Intervals in combination with circuit training, either by putting intervals within your circuit program or by having intervals as a separate cardio workout, bring great fat loss results. Whatever the case, the ultimate in fat burning results. Circuit training is very efficient because you are able to work several different components of fitness, i.e., strength, endurance, and flexibility. Our circuit training system is divided into a beginner's circuit, an intermediate circuit, and an advanced circuit.

The beginner's circuit is a lower intensity level through the manipulation of time of circuit, exercise difficulty, and rest periods. For example, exercises are less explosive than in the advanced circuit, and bodyweight exercises are done without movement, such as bear crawls and crab walks, where not only stabilizing bodyweight is necessary but moving bodyweight forward or backwards is also required. Workouts also have more rest periods. Overall, the beginner's circuit is an easier workout, from type of exercise to the intensity level specified.

Intermediate circuit workouts are a stepping stone to advanced workouts. The rest periods are shorter and exercises are more intense than in beginner circuits. The bodyweight exercises are more taxing and require more balance and coordination. Advanced workouts are perfect for somebody who is experienced and accustomed to high intensity workouts. Also, for somebody who has gone through the beginning workouts for four to five weeks and the intermediate workouts for four to five weeks.

The advanced circuit has high intensity bodyweight movements and explosive type of dumbbell movements that will definitely challenge you. The advanced programs are designed to be very intense, using short rest periods, grouping exercises and very high repetitions, and timed exercises that go as long as one minute in duration.

Will Lifting Weights Bulk Me Up?

Will lifting weights bulk me up? I hear this question many times, mostly from women. (It's alright; I'm not mad at you.) Most of the women who ask me about bulking up know someone who started an exercise program—usually on her own—and gained weight. Rest assured that the weight gain was not from strength training. The only reason she got bigger was from what she was doing at the dinner table. A strength training program will put muscle on your body. That's what it's supposed to do. Muscle is metabolically active tissue and will elevate your metabolism. An elevated metabolism should be a top priority for somebody in pursuit of fat loss. A faster metabolism will burn body fat whether you're watching television, working out or sleeping. The long-term answer to the metabolism question is strength training. Where people go wrong is that they elevate their metabolism from strength training, thereby increasing their appetites. However, instead of eating nutritious food, they continue with bad eating habits and consuming fat and simple carbohydrates—a recipe for disaster.

What happens to people who put on fat at the same time they put on muscle? They get bulky. There is no physiological way that a woman who just started an exercise program could put on muscle at a rate that would result in her being viewed as bulky from muscle mass. The culprit: Diet.

Her new-found bulkiness has nothing to do with strength training. Strength training did its job; she just has to cooperate and eat correctly. Consider what someone who has been training for years would think when she hears a beginner complaining that she is getting too bulky. People who have been training for years, struggling for every bit of muscle fiber they can build, hears a beginner complain about gaining too muscle and laughs. Once the beginner puts on fat along with muscle and experiences some bulkiness, discouragement sets in and she automatically wants to quit. What the beginner, or anyone for that matter, has to understand about starting a strength training program and accelerating her metabolism—thus increasing her appetite—is that she needs to consume nutritious food. Weight training alone will not "bulk" her up. Eating junk food will.

Is Lifting Weights Safe?

Lifting weights is by far one of the safest activities you can partake in during the course of a day. Weightlifters who lift incredible amounts of weight at amazing speeds have very low incidences of injuries. A study done by Brian Hamill in 1994 compared incidences of injury in over ten sports, including rugby, basketball, football, gymnastics, tennis, power lifting, squash, volleyball, cross country, and school-aged soccer. He found the safest sport to be weightlifting, with 0.0018 injuries per 100 participation hours.

Considering that obesity is at pandemic levels, I believe that a lack of training is more dangerous than not participating in a weightlifting program. What are some of the "benefits" to look forward to with a sedentary lifestyle? Oh, I don't know, maybe diabetes, high blood pressure, and heart disease, to name a few. There are many activities in life that if done carelessly can lead to accidents. Driving a car can lead to serious trouble if you aren't paying attention to the road. Riding a bike can lead to major difficulties if you aren't paying attention to traffic. The same thing goes for lifting weights. If you aren't paying attention and are just going through the motions, then obviously injuries can happen.

In this day and age, it is imperative that we engage in a fitness program. Everyday life seems to be less and less physically challenging. Gone are the days of physical labor to make ends meet, or strenuous labor and chores around the house for maintenance purposes; these jobs are now performed by other people. This e-book and will provide

you with all the instruction you'll need to be successful and
to achieve your fitness goals.

Getting Started

Getting started in an exercise program can be an intimidating and daunting task, but it doesn't have to be. This e-book gives you a list of great fat-burning, muscle-building exercises. You also have descriptions, pictures, and programs of how to do the exercises correctly and safely. In addition, you can perform these exercises in the comfort of your own home. You don't have to go to a crowded gym and wait for someone to finish with the dumbbells you need. At home, you can bypass all of the crowds; all you need are some dumbbells, barbells, and your bodyweight, for an incredible workout.

Have a Starting Point

Let's make sure we have a starting point. Using several different measurement methods is the best way to chart your progress and see all the improvements that you will make over the next several months. Take pictures of yourself from several angles—front, side, and back. Keep your arms to your side and wear a bathing suit or another outfit that clearly outlines your body.

Have a fitness trainer take your body fat measurements for free at a local gym. They should have calipers or an electrical impedance mechanism to take these measurements. Repeat these measurements every four weeks to ensure that you are on the right track and to determine whether you need to adjust the nutritional or training program, such as increasing or decreasing calories or increasing the intensity of your workouts. Consistent measurements will help you stay on track towards your goals.

Also, take measurements of your waist, hips, legs, and arms. These measurements show—in black and white—the inches coming off your body. Remember that sometimes the scale won't show the fat loss because of an increase in muscle. This makes the measuring tape a valuable asset.

Do weigh yourself, but if your measurements are decreasing and your clothes are fitting better yet your weight hasn't moved, then you know you have put on muscle. On the flip side, if your weight is dropping rapidly by more than four to five pounds per week, and you are also feeling tired and burned out, you could be losing weight too rapidly and have begun to lose muscle—the opposite of our goals. At this point, the scale serves as a great indicator that you need to increase your caloric intake and work on putting some muscle back on, thereby increasing your energy level.

Metabolism

Recent studies have found that, contrary to what was believed, a pound of muscle does not burn 50 calories a day. The actual number of calories that muscle burns per day is about six. Although studies have determined this lower amount, the fact still remains the same—the more muscle you have, the more calories you will burn. In fact, although fat was thought to be calorically inactive, it actually burns two calories per hour. Nevertheless, fat is not what we want on our bodies.

Determining your resting metabolic rate (RMR) is realistic because it gives a better idea of one's actual metabolic rate. This measurement is taken while you are awake and your muscles are active, as opposed to your basal metabolic rate (BMR), which is measured while lying down and completely at rest, and as if asleep. For example, when determining your RMR, the small muscles of your face are contracting, the muscles of your body are working to sit you up straight, and other cellular functions are occurring to make this measurement much more applicable. The number of calories burned will be about 5% to 15% more than that indicated by your BMR. This indicates that all functions of the body, no matter how small, contribute to one's overall caloric expenditure.

There is something called excess post-exercise oxygen consumption (EPOC). EPOC is the amount of energy expended from your body after a workout that is used to restore your body to the pre-exercise condition. This means that even after a workout, your body is still burning calories for you.

Research suggests that exercise should be high intensity (strength training) and short in duration (interval training), the opposite of L.S.D. (long slow distance), which we covered earlier in the book. EPOC is optimized through short bouts of high intensity training (strength training). Strength training bodes well for people with time restrictions and who have a hard time carving out hour after hour for aerobic training. Strength training not only burns the most fat, it does so in the shortest time. Starting a strength training program will bring higher energy output from not only the actual workout itself, but also from the recovery after the workout.

Nutrition

The Ultimate Women's Fat Loss System nutritional program is based on healthy eating for life instead of on the temporary approach of dieting. As I mentioned earlier, there are no stones unturned; mastering the fundamentals of healthy eating for a lifetime is what works.

There are literally countless diets on the market, "the flavor of the month," so to speak, all guaranteeing to bring weight loss in record time. You have seen the ads—"30lbs in 30 days"—splashed across the headlines of the latest gossip magazine. What are these diets really about? Are they dropping calories dangerously low, which, in the long term, wrecks your metabolism and causes other physiological problems? Don't get me wrong, there are successful nutritional programs out there. I'm just giving you what has worked for my clients for the last fifteen years. There are no shortcuts, magic foods, or macronutrient breakdowns that will bring magical results without the discipline and desire to want to change your body and your life. It's all about the basic foods that are available to everyone who wants to burn fat.

Meal Frequency

Yes, you must eat small, frequent meals throughout the day. This may seem counterproductive but eating frequently during the day, preferably every three to four hours, will actually speed the fat loss process. If you think logically, eating more to weigh less makes no sense, but it is essential if fat loss is a part of your goal.

If you restrict your food intake to one meal per day, your body screams, "You haven't fed me. I'm storing calories as fat." In essence, the less food you eat, the more fat you put on.

Additionally, eating one big meal a day increases your insulin levels, making it difficult to burn fat as energy because of the abundance of sugar in the blood. As a result, your body stores fat. Essentially, you could have two people eat the same amount of calories. One person consumes his or her calories at one sitting and the other eats small, frequent meals throughout the day. The person who eats small meals throughout the day will be successful at fat loss because less glucose is in her bloodstream, which means less insulin is released. When insulin is on an even keel, the body is more apt to store glucose as glycogen and not pack it away as fat in fat cells.

Many people try extreme diets, thinking that fewer calories are better. However, the opposite is true.

When this happens, the body hoards calories and one's metabolism slows to a screeching stop. One of the keys to fat loss is reducing calories gradually, by approximately 10% to 15%. As I have already stated, this will ensure that the body doesn't go into starvation mode. For example, if your normal caloric intake is 3,000 calories, take in 2,700 calories to initiate fat loss. If you want to be a bit more aggressive, you can reduce your calories by 15% to bring your caloric intake to 2,550. The main point is to decrease your caloric intake enough to initiate some fat loss but not to the point where your body senses a dramatic caloric loss and inhibits fat from being used as energy. You must have the energy to perform your daily tasks. If your energy levels are down, you will be more apt to go off your nutritional plan with a quick energy source, such as simple carbohydrates like candy or cookies. In turn, this will throw your insulin levels out of whack and instigate a vicious circle—with gaining fat as the result.

Insulin Resistance

Insulin resistance is initiated by several unhealthy contributors, the worst being trans fats. The outer layer of the muscle cell serves as the receptor site for insulin. When this outer layer is damaged, glucose gathers in the bloodstream and the pancreas pumps out insulin. This scenario leads to significant fat storage in the body.

The leading contributors to insulin resistance are elevated sugar levels, lack of exercise, stress, smoking, and alcohol. If conditions are good, insulin binds with muscle, and glucose is stored as glycogen and used by the muscles as energy.

Insulin Sensitivity

Strength training, along with a diet that includes lean forms of protein, fruits, and vegetables (fiber) can change receptors from being resistant to insulin to being sensitive to insulin. Strength training utilizes glucose as energy, and with continued exercise, the muscles will store more glucose in the form of glycogen as fuel for workouts.

As you increase your training loads, the cell receptors on muscle tissue are more prone to welcoming insulin and glucose, meaning more glucose in your muscles and less in the bloodstream. That said, a decrease in insulin levels ensures that fat is utilized as energy instead of stored in fat cells.

Omega-3 fatty acids help to reverse the destructive effects on muscle cells that sugar, trans fats, alcohol, and stress bring. You can find Omega-3 fatty acids in fish that carry a larger proportion of fat, such as sardines, salmon, mackerel, trout, and eel. Studies have conclusively shown that populations consuming large amounts of cold water fish and other northern marine animals have lower instances of diabetes than other populations in other places in the world. Omega-3 fatty acids increase insulin sensitivity, and the body in turn releases less insulin, stores less fat, and insulin is allowed to do its job, which is to get carbohydrates and amino acids into muscle tissue.

Omega-3 fatty acids have also been found to reduce

stickiness on your platelets (the cells circulating in the blood that are involved in the cellular mechanisms of primary hemostasis). Moreover, Omega-3 fatty acids can lower triglycerides by 65%. Elevated triglycerides are linked to high blood pressure, kidney failure, stroke, and heart attack.

Carbohydrates and Insulin

Carbohydrate conversations are hot nowadays. Everywhere you look, there are diets claiming that low carbs are best, or that high carbs are best. Deciding which way to go, as you know, can be a difficult task.

There are two types of carbohydrates: complex and simple. Complex carbohydrates are healthier. There are two forms of complex carbohydrates: fibrous and starchy. Both are unprocessed and are slowly released into the bloodstream, which ensures low insulin levels.

Carbohydrates, whether simple or complex, convert to a sugar in the blood called glucose. As mentioned earlier, the difference between simple carbohydrates and complex carbohydrates is the rate at which each type is broken down.

Complex carbohydrates are broken down at a much slower rate because they are unprocessed; this creates more work for the body and initiates balanced energy levels, as opposed to the peaks and valleys commonly experienced with simple carbohydrates. Simple carbohydrates are in the foods that most of us love but know we shouldn't, such as candy, cookies, cakes, ice cream, sodas—basically, the full array of junk food.

To ensure that the body works efficiently, it strives for balance by keeping blood sugar levels between 70–110 mgs of glucose. If the blood sugar level gets close to 110 mgs or goes beyond it, the pancreas releases insulin. Insulin takes the sugar out of the blood and shuttles it to muscle or fat cells, lowering glucose levels in the to the 70–110 mgs range. If blood sugar levels fall below 70 mgs, the body releases glucagon, which takes sugar out of muscle tissue and puts it into the bloodstream. You will notice that these two hormones, glucagon and insulin, work together to keep blood sugar levels between 70 mgs and 110 mgs.

The discussion of glucagon and insulin enhances the importance of consuming balanced meals. Eating a meal consisting of only carbohydrates elevates insulin levels, which we already know isn't the best situation for achieving fat loss goals. Consuming a balanced meal consisting of a protein and a carbohydrate will result in a combined release of glucagon and insulin, which means that your insulin level will not go through the roof. The presence of protein ensures that the pancreas releases glucagon and, in turn, lowers insulin levels.

Fat

There are several forms of fat, all of which have nine calories per gram, in comparison to carbohydrates and protein, which put out four calories per gram. The body has a much easier time digesting fat than it does protein and carbohydrates. You can see why fat has received a bad rap. From 100 calories of fat, the body can use 97 calories. With 100 calories of protein, the body can use 80 calories, and with 100 calories of carbohydrates, the body can use 90 calories.

The first form of fat that I will review is saturated fat, which is found in animal sources. Saturated fats are solid at room temperature. For health reasons, saturated fat consumption should be limited. However, if you are consuming animal products as a lean source of protein, completely avoiding saturated fats is impossible.

The second form of fat is monounsaturated fat, which should make up a good portion of your fat intake. The most popular monounsaturated fat is olive oil.

The third form of fat is trans fatty acids, probably the worst of the bunch. Trans fatty acids are man-made and found in all processed foods. Avoid trans fats like the plague.

The fourth and last form of fat is polyunsaturated fats, also known as essential fatty acids. These are Omega-6 and Omega-3 fatty acids. Omega-6 fatty acids are abundant in our diet while Omega-3 sources are not. As we've already talked about, consuming an Omega-3 source is important, and you can do this by taking a fish capsule or flax seed oil, or by eating fish such as salmon, sardines, and herring.

Fiber

Fiber is a very important aspect in the fat loss riddle. You've probably heard that you should eat your vegetables. Whoever said this to you had the best intentions for you in mind, because he or she was basically telling you, in a roundabout way, to eat your fiber.

Fiber has many health benefits, such as reducing fat levels and lowering the risk of diabetes and heart disease. Sources of fiber include fruits, vegetables, and grains. Fiber, also known as roughage or bulk, also includes sections of plant foods that the body doesn't digest. Fiber is different from protein, carbohydrates, and fat, which the body absorbs and digests. Fiber moves through your body (stomach, small intestine) and into your colon undigested.

There are two types of fiber. Insoluble fiber dissolves in water and soluble fiber does not dissolve in water. Insoluble fiber enhances the movement of food through the digestive system. Soluble fiber melts into liquid to form a gel-like substance. This gel-like substance aids in decreasing levels of cholesterol and glucose in the blood.

For good reason, fiber is also looked upon as a fat-reducing asset because of the energy needed to absorb fat. The body has a difficult task in breaking down the vegetables you consume, and actually dispenses energy to digest these contents. This means that eating your vegetables gives your body the ability to lower your cholesterol and glucose levels, and burn calories. Your mom was right all along—eat your vegetables!

<u>Protein</u>

Protein is a very important aspect of your nutritional plan. The other macronutrients are also needed, but protein is arguably the most important. Protein comes from animal sources such as chicken, fish, turkey, meat, egg whites, and dairy. These forms of protein are all complete forms, meaning that each one contains all of the essential amino acids, also known as the building blocks of protein.

Protein from non-animal sources is called incomplete protein. Incomplete proteins lack one or more of the essential amino acids. Complete proteins are broken down into amino acids in the same fashion that carbohydrates are broken down into glucose.

Protein also kicks into gear the hormone glucagon. Glucagon tweaks the fat-storing potential of high insulin levels and kicks the fat burning process into gear, separating fatty acids from fat cells.

Protein is difficult for the body to digest, which means that your body does not assimilate all of the calories that you consume, because calories are burned while digesting protein. For example, when you eat 300 calories of lean red meat, the body is effective at holding on to 80% of all 300 calories, which means that you actually use 240 calories of the original 300. The body uses the other 60 calories to help digest the lean red meat. Essentially, food provides energy for basic functions and daily tasks, and the body also spends energy burning food.

Calorie Restrictions

Restrict your caloric intake by no more than 10% to 15% below your normal maintenance levels. There are several ways to figure out your normal caloric intake, but first we must figure out the number of calories you need just to sustain life at total rest.

To be more exact, figure out your body fat percentage with skin calipers. This will help you determine the amount of fat and muscle you have on your body. For example, if you weigh 160 pounds and your body fat measures 20%, your body is 80% muscle. Weighing 160 pounds with 20% fat means that you have 32 pounds of fat and 128 pounds of lean muscle mass on your body.

Therefore, to sustain life at complete rest, you need to consume 1,280 calories (128 pounds of lean muscle mass x 10) a day. As discussed earlier, this is your RMR, or the number of calories you need to sustain your muscle mass and get energy to your vital organs and your brain.

If you go below your RMR, you are asking for trouble. If you drop below your RMR, your body will start to burn muscle mass as energy and take amino acids from your organs to survive. Essentially, your body will decrease its muscle mass, which slows your metabolism. Instead of achieving fat loss from reduced calories, the body learns to function on less and gains weight.

I'm sure that you have heard people say, "I don't know why I can't lose weight. I hardly eat anything. I should be losing weight." Therein lies the problem; the body has been conditioned to survive on less calories, meaning less muscle mass and slower metabolism.

Muscle loss also affects insulin maintenance and increases insulin resistance. The insulin receptors on your muscles decrease, leaving insulin to gather in the bloodstream and glucose to be shuttled to fat cells.

What Are My Calorie Requirements?

To find out how many calories you need, we'll use as an example a 160 pound person with 20% body fat and 128 pounds of lean body mass. We calculate the 128 pounds of lean body mass as follows:

1. 160 pounds with 20% body fat, or 160 x .20 = 32 pounds of body fat
2. 160 pounds – 32 pounds of body fat = 128 pounds of lean body mass

Previously, we discussed the number of calories needed to sustain life with absolutely no activity. Now, let's determine the number of calories needed to perform daily tasks such as work, fitness training, errands, and other intense activities. Previously, we determined that one's RMR was 1,280 calories. Now, RMR for a more active lifestyle can be calculated as:

RMR: 1,280 calories x 1 + RMR = 2,560 calories. Basically, you have doubled your RMR as a result of being physically active.

The following equations can be used to determine different levels of RMR, based on level of activity:

Intense Activity: RMR x 1 + RMR
Very Active: RMR x .7 + RMR
Moderate Activity:RMR x .4 + RMR
No Activity: RMR x .2 + RMR

A pound of fat equals 3,500 calories. Therefore, to lose a pound of fat in a way that spares muscle mass, you must ensure that you are losing 1.5–2 pounds a week. However, reducing your intake by 3,500 calories a week isn't always the right answer. Remember the 10– 15% restriction on reducing your caloric intake to prevent your body from using up your muscle mass for energy. So, let's consider a situation where reducing your caloric intake by 3,500 calories a week could be excessive and may consequently lead to metabolic shutdown.

Suppose you're consuming 2,000 calories a day and decide to lose a pound of fat per week. Seems like an achievable and painless goal; however, applying the 3,500 calorie = 1 pound of fat rule implies a daily reduction of 500 calories. This is a drastic reduction in calories of 25% (500 / 2,000 = 25%), which will lead to metabolic slowdown because your body is burning up muscle to get enough energy, simultaneous with losing fat. Muscle, the machinery that burns fat, is being wasted in the process.

Remember, if you reduce your calories by 10 to 15% you might not lose your goal of a pound of fat a week; however, rest assured that your improvements will be steady and consistent, and you'll protect your muscles, ensuring fat loss, inches lost, and continued success.

Nutritional Plan

To ensure rapid yet healthy fat loss, your eating plan will consist of balanced meals, protein, complex carbohydrates, and healthy fats. Let's first determine how many grams of protein you will need per day. You'll need one gram of protein per pound of lean body mass. Some might say that's not enough, or maybe too much, protein but I believe that figuring out your lean body mass, as we did earlier, will give you an accurate starting point for your protein needs and a great starting point to initiate your fat-burning, muscle-building nutritional plan.

With our plan, you eat fibrous and unprocessed carbohydrates in the form of vegetables and fruits. We also use starchy, unprocessed sources of carbohydrates, but timed so that you consume them either at the beginning of the day, giving you time to burn them off, or after workouts, when your muscles are depleted and ready to vacuum in the carbohydrates that you just ate to replenish glycogen stores.

Cheat meals, or free meals as I would rather have you call them, begin four weeks into the program. I want to make sure you're on the right track before we introduce foods that got you into trouble in the past. Don't worry; after four weeks we will put those foods back in. More on that later.

Here are a few examples of meals. For breakfast, you can have egg whites (protein), oatmeal (complex carbohydrate), and a handful of nuts (healthy fats). An early morning snack may consist of two slices of string cheese, a green apple, and pecans. Lunch will be a turkey wrap with a piece of fruit and a handful of walnuts. Your mid-afternoon snack may consist of cottage cheese, sliced strawberries, and some macadamia nuts. And, for dinner, have grilled chicken breast, salad, and some asparagus. With that, you will have five balanced and very nutritious meals to get your metabolism working and help you burn body fat. We'll present more meal ideas just ahead.

Remember that eating multiple meals helps keep insulin levels on an even keel. They also require energy to digest the food you've eaten. Either way, eating small, frequent, and balanced meals burns body fat and brings you closer to your fat loss goals.

Grocery Shopping

One of the most important things that you can do for yourself regarding grocery shopping is to avoid going when you're hungry. This is a recipe for disaster. Starving and shopping is a bad combination. Have something nutritious before you head down to the supermarket. Consume protein, such as yogurt or cottage cheese, or anything that takes the edge off while you're at the store. I'm sure you've heard this before: stay to the outside aisles as much as possible, as the middle of the store can be deadly. Sure, the middle aisles display some essentials there, but serious transgressions can happen there. Make a list of the items you came to pick up so you're not wandering aimlessly around the store. Have a list, get what you need, and get out.

One last thing. Make sure you read the labels of the items you're buying. You might think you're buying something that is supposed to have no carbohydrates, yet you later find out that it was loaded with carbohydrates. Please read the labels.

The following are foods in certain food categories, including their calorie, protein, and fat counts.

Sources of Protein

	Calories	Protein	Fat	Carbohydrates
Flank steak, 3.5 oz	263	27.0	16.4	0
Sirloing steak, 3.5oz	229	29.2	11.6	0
Ground extra lean beef, 3.5 oz	256	25.4	16.3	0
Tuna, white, canned in water, 3 oz	109	20.1	20.5	0
Halibut, baked, 3 oz	119	22.7	2.5	0
Orange roughly, baked, 3 oz	76	16.0	0.8	0
Egg, white only, 1 large	17	3.5	0	0.3
Egg, scrambled, 1 large	93	6.3	7.0	0.6
Cottage cheese, fat-free 1 cup	160	30.0	0	10.0
Turkey breast 1 slice	23	4.7	0.3	0
Mozzarella, string, 1 oz stick	80	7.0	6.0	1,0
Chicken breast, half roasted	142	26.7	3.1	0

Sources of Carbohydrates

	Calories	Protein	Fat	Carbohydrates
Sweet potato, baked	117	2.0	0.1	27.7
Potato, baked with skin	220	4.6	0.2	51.0
Apple, raw, 1 medium	81	0.3	0.5	21.0
Oats, dry, 100% rolled, ½ cup	150	5.0	3.0	3.0
Multigrain bread, 1 slice	65	3.0	1.0	12.0
Wild rice, boiled, 1 cup	170	7.0	1.0	35.0
Multigrain, Quaker, ½ cup	133	4.5	1.0	29.4
Nutrigrain wheat, ¾ cup	100	3.0	1.0	24.0
Blueberries, raw, 1 cup	81	1.0	0.6	20.5
Guava, raw, 1 cup	46	0.7	0.5	10.7
Strawberries, raw, 1 cup	45	0.9	0.6	10.5

Sources of Fat

	Calories	Protein	Fat	Carbohydrates
Almonds, 1 oz	166	4.6	14.6	6.9
Macadameia nuts, 1oz	200	2.5	21.1	3.2
Sunflower seeds, no shell, 1 oz	165	5.5	14.1	6.8
Avacado, 1 medium	306	3.7	30.0	12.0
Walnuts, dried, 1 oz	190	4.0	19.9	4.0
Olive oil, 1 Tbs	124	0	14.0	0

Sample Meals

The following are a few sample meal plans that are balanced with a protein, a carbohydrate, and a healthy fat. You can adjust the calories for your specific goals and needs. You are only limited by your imagination; just make it healthy, and have fun!

Breakfast		
1 cup non fat cottage cheese 1 cup strawberries 1 oz walnuts	1 stick string cheese 3 egg whites, ½ cup grapes ½ cup strawberries 1 oz walnuts	¼ cups oatmeal in water 4 oz nonfat cottage cheese 1 orange 1 oz pecans
Protein: 34, Carb: 25, Fat: 19 Total Calories: 395	Protein: 20, Carb: 41, Fat: 27 Total Calories: 487	Protein: 27, Carb: 26, Fat: 23 Total Calories: 419
Midmorning Snack		
1 slice turkey breast 1 slice lettuce wrap 2 Tbsp guacamole 1 slice tomato	1 cup nonfat cottage cheese 1 banana 1 oz almonds	1 hard-boiled egg 1 string cheese 1 tangerine ¼ cup almonds
Protein: 6, Carb: 3, Fat: 5 Total Calories: 73	Protein: 30, Carb: 44, Fat: 15 Total Calories: 431	Protein: 19, Carb: 17, Fat: 28 Total Calories: 396
Lunch		
Chicken breast sandwich 3.5 oz chicken breast, g1rilled 2 slices rye bread 1 TbspDionna-se 1 lettuce leaf tomato slice 1oz walnuts	Tuna salad sandwhich 2 slices whole wheat bread 3 oz water packed tuna 1 Tbsp canola mayonnaise ¼ chopped onions ¼ tomato slice 1 lettuce leaf	3.5 oz flank steak ¼ avocado sliced sliced tomatoes whole wheat tortilla

Protein: 31, Carb: 35, Fat: 21 Total Calories: 453	Protein: 20, Carb: 23, Fat: 11 Total Calories: 271	Protein: 30, Carb: 19, Fat: 5 Total Calories: 421
Mid-afternoon Snack		
1 cup non fat yogurt 1 oz sunflower seeds 1 cup strawberries	1 stiick string cheese 1 green apple ¼ cup almonds	1 orange 2 Tbsp peanut butter ¼ cup almonds
Protein: 15, Carb: 35, Fat: 14 Total Calories: 337	Protein: 11, Carb: 28, Fat: 15 Total Calories: 291	Protein: 14, Carb: 22, Fat: 31 Total Calories: 423
Dinner		
3.5 oz top sirloin steamed asparagus large salad w/ balsamic and olive oil dressing	3.5 oz chicken breast grilled vegietables large- tossed green salad 2 Tbsp oil/vinegar dressing	4 oz salmon 1 cup brown rice 1 cup spinach
Protein: 29, Carb: 5, Fat: 26 Total Calories: 370	Protein: 27, Carb: 10, Fat: 5 Total Calories: 193	Protein: 37, Carb: 44, Fat: 6 Total Calories: 378
Total Daily Calories= 1,628	**Total Daily Calories= 1,673**	**Total Daily Calories= 2,037**

Breakfast		
3 scrambled whole eggs 2 slices wheat toast w/ butter ½ grapefruit	1 cup nonfat yogurt 1 cup strawberries ¼ cup pecans ½ cantaloupe	3 egg whites 1 whole egg scrambled 1 whole wheat tortilla ¼ cup walnuts
Protein: 29, Carb: 5, Fat: 26 Total Calories: 411	Protein: 15, Carb: 35, Fat: 21 Total Calories: 389	Protein: 21, Carb: 20, Fat: 30 Total Calories: 434
Midmorning Snack		
¼ cup almonds 1 banana	2 Tbsp peanut butter 1 apple cut in slices	1 cup nonfat yogurt 1 cup blueberries ¼ cup almonds
Protein: 7, Carb: 32, Fat: 15 Total Calories: 291	Protein: 9, Carb: 25, Fat: 16 Total Calories: 276	Protein: 19, Carb: 43, Fat: 15 Total Calories: 379
Lunch		
3.5 oz ground turkey breast burger ½ avocado 2 slices rye bread 1 lettuce leaf 1 slice tomato	3.5 oz chicken breast 1 slice tomato ¼ cup walnuts ½ avocado sliced ½. cup alfalfa sprouts	3.5 oz steak fajita ½ avocado onions bell peppers salsa fat free sour cream 1 whole wheat tortilla
Protein: 33, Carb: 34, Fat: 5 Total Calories: 313	Protein: 36, Carb: 6, Fat: 26 Total Calories: 402	Protein: 19, Carb: 21, Fat: 21 Total Calories: 389

<table>
<tr><th colspan="3">Mid-afternoon Snack</th></tr>
<tr>
<td>1 cup nonfat cottage cheese

1 pear

¼ cup sliced almonds</td>
<td>1 stick string cheese

1 small salad

¼ cup sunflower seeds

¼ cup walnuts</td>
<td>½ whole wheat bagel

½ cup nonfat cottage cheese</td>
</tr>
<tr>
<td>Protein: 25, Carb: 28, Fat: 15

Total Calories: 347</td>
<td>Protein: 17, Carb: 11, Fat: 32

Total Calories: 400</td>
<td>Protein: 17, Carb: 23, Fat: 1

Total Calories: 169</td>
</tr>
<tr><th colspan="3">Dinner</th></tr>
<tr>
<td>4 oz orange roughly

1 cup spinach

1 cup wild rice</td>
<td>3.5 oz pork chop broiled

1 cup green beans

1 large potato, whipped butter</td>
<td>3.5 oz grilled halibut

1 cup brussel sprouts

large salad

1 Tbsp olive oil

2 Tbsp balsamic vinegar</td>
</tr>
<tr>
<td>Protein: 15, Carb: 35, Fat: 1

Total Calories: 209</td>
<td>Protein: 28, Carb: 64, Fat: 18

Total Calories: 530</td>
<td>Protein: 22, Carb: 3, Fat: 21

Total Calories: 289</td>
</tr>
<tr>
<td>Total Daily Calories= 1,571</td>
<td>Total Daily Calories= 1,997</td>
<td>Total Daily Calories= 1,660</td>
</tr>
</table>

Free Meals

A free meal, or a cheat meal, whatever you choose to call it, will benefit you psychologically more than anything else. You aren't really cheating so I don't want you to feel guilty and go back to eating cheeseburgers and fries—not when we've come this far. Don't worry, it's a meal you have earned for being good for five days. Yes, I said five days. You get two free meals that you can have on nonconsecutive days. One of the meals should be on the weekend, and the other on a weekday, which will help you avoid being a total pain in the butt with a restricted diet when going out with friends or a significant other during the weekend.

Your cheat meal should consist of the foods that you have been craving the most. If you've been craving pizza, have some pizza, but don't have the whole pizza. Eat a meal, not the entire buffet. The purpose of this meal is to take the edge off dieting and give you a chance to taste some of the foods that you have been thinking most about. These two meals aren't going to pack on fat and, more importantly, they will help you stick to your eating plan for the long term because knowing a free meal is coming within days helps ease the stress of a diet and brings some flexibility to your eating routine.

I would like you to include a protein source with your free meals to help control your insulin levels and keep your blood sugar on an even keel. In addition, you won't be able to eat as much of the bad stuff if you have protein.

Just remember not to turn your free meals into a

contest to see how much you can eat. Have a sensible, well-portioned meal and, again, enjoy some of the foods that you have been craving.

One more thing. Don't worry about a slight weight gain after your free meal. You may experience some water retention from the carbohydrates that you eat, so wait three or four days after your free meal before you weigh in again.

Water

Water is a very important component to not only your nutritional program but to living a healthy life. Water is the most abundant substance in your body, helps to cool your body after strenuous exercise, aids with digestion and aids in lubricating your joints. Your goal is to drink half your bodyweight in ounces. If you weigh 150 pounds, your goal is to drink 75 ounces of water per day. This is a difficult goal to achieve but keeping a water bottle with you at all times will help you drink water throughout the day and stay hydrated. If you do this, you will definitely see a difference in how you feel and look.

Condiments

Salad is usually a positive choice for your diet. However, if you smother your salad in ranch dressing, you are ruining your meal. Put salad dressing on the side and dip into it. Stay away from white sauces and ketchup (loaded with sugar). Instead, use spices, salsa, mustard, and vinaigrette dressings. If you use soy sauce, choose the low-sodium version, and use the low-fat version of mayonnaise. Salsa is versatile and can be used on salads, baked potato, and other items.

Organic Food

When it comes to the food industry, there seems to be a well-debated issue of Organic vs. Non-Organic food. What's the difference? Is there a difference? Why is one pear exactly twice as much money at the grocery store than another... Are these designer pears we're dealing with here?

The truth is that Organic farming has been around for a very long time. As American agriculture grew as an industry, so did output needs which led (ironically enough) to more industrialized farming techniques, cheaper shortcuts, and more mass farming. The effects to not only our population's health, but to our planet have been felt since then... And some of us (call us old-fashioned) are heading back to smaller, natural farming... The way they used to do it in the old days.

There are a whole host of reasons why people buy and cook organically. Many of which we'll explore here. Basically, it all boils down to the adage of: "You are what you eat." -Some of us prefer to be Organic.

What is Organic Food?

There is a great deal of misunderstanding surrounding what IS and what is NOT **organic** food. To begin with, let's start with the term **"organic"** and what it actually means. When a food is described as being **"organic,"** what we're referring to is not the actual food itself, but rather refers to the way in which the food is processed. **Organic** food is farmed and processed without the use of pesticides, antibiotics, preservatives, irradiation, or genetically modified organisms.

Organic agriculture, it stands to reason, is based on a replenishment system of farming that maintains soil fertility without the use of often toxic pesticides and persistent fertilizers.

On October 21, 2002, the United States Department of Agriculture's (USDA) National Organic Program (NOP) established a set of clear guidelines to ensure consumer awareness of organic content in purchased food.

Before we delve into what goes behind the USDA Organic label, let's take a look at the varying classifications of "organic" foods.

Classifications of Organic Food

It is important to note that although there are several classifications of **organic** food, only those that constitute 95% or more **organic** ingredients can earn the USDA "**organic**" seal of approval.

100% Organic —Foods made with 100% **organic** ingredients; no synthetic ingredients whatsoever. May display the USDA **Organic** seal.

Organic—Products containing at least 95% **organic** ingredients; remaining ingredients are not available organically but are NOP approved. May display the USDA **Organic** seal.

Made With Organic Ingredient s— Foods containing at least 70% **organic** ingredients. Not eligible for the USDA **Organic** seal.

Sometimes eggs, meat, poultry, and dairy products are labeled "**organic**". According to USDA Regulations, that requires that the farm animals these products are derived from have never received either antibiotics or genetically modified growth hormones. **Organic** meat is therefore extremely hard to find.

What are the Basic Requirements for Organic Certification?

The USDA developed The National Organic Program Final Rule (NOP) to implement the Organic Foods Production Act of 1990 (OFPA). The NOP was founded based upon recommendations by the National Organic Standards Board (NOSB), appointed by the Secretary of Agriculture. The NOSB was instituted to implement OFPA and to review substances permitted for organic production and handling.

Now that's what I call a mouthful!

Basically, all **organic** certifiers who operate, sell, OR certify products sold as **"organic"** in the United States must be accredited by the USDA according to specific guidelines set forth, which we will cover shortly.

For the record, it cannot be stressed enough that **"organic"** describes the processing and handling of **organic** food, more so than it does the actual food product itself. This is very important to keep in mind, as later we tackle the questions of nutrition and cost in the **organic** market placce.

"Organic production" is defined by the regulation as "a production system that is managed ... to respond to site-specific conditions by integrating cultural, biological, and mechanical practices that foster cycling of resources, promote ecological balance, and conserve biodiversity."[1]

The Organic Ecology website features a very long, completely comprehensive summary of the USDA National Organic Program Final Rule. (Written by Jim Riddle, UMN, and Miles McEvoy, Washington State Department of Agriculture.)[2]

NOP Regulations for Organic Labeling

For our purposes here, the NOP regulations for **Organic** labeling require:

<u>For crop farms:</u>

- 3 years with no application of prohibited materials (no synthetic fertilizers, pesticides, or GMOs) prior to harvest of the first certified organic crop Implementation of an Organic System Plan, with proactive fertility systems; conservation measures; environmentally sound manure, weed, disease, and pest management practices; and soil building crop rotation systems

- Use of natural inputs and/or approved synthetic substances on the National List;

- No use of prohibited substances while certified;

- No use of genetically engineered organisms, (GMOs) defined in the rule as "excluded methods"

- No sewage sludge or irradiation;

- Use of organic seeds, when commercially available

- Use of organic seedlings for annual crops

- Restrictions on use of raw manure and compost

- Maintenance of buffer zones, depending on risk of contamination

- No residues of prohibited substances exceeding 5% of the EPA tolerance.

<u>For livestock operations:</u>

- Implementation of an Organic Livestock Plan;

- Mandatory outdoor access, when seasonally appropriate

- Access to pasture for ruminants

- No antibiotics, growth hormones, slaughter byproducts, or GMOs

- 100% organic feed and approved feed supplements

- Sound animal husbandry and preventative health care

- Organic management from last third of gestation or 2nd day after hatching

- No rotating animals between organic and non-organic management.

<u>For processing operations:</u>

- No commingling or contamination of organic products during processing

- Implementation of an Organic Handling Plan

- No use of GMOs or irradiation

- Proactive sanitation and facility pest management practices

- Use of organic agricultural ingredients in "organic" products, when commercially available

- Use of approved label claims for "100% organic", "organic" (at least 95% organic ingredients), "Made with organic ingredients" (at least 70% organic ingredients), and proper use of the word "organic" in ingredient list (less than 70% organic ingredients)[3]

Who Regulates Certified Organic Claims?

The Organic Food Production Act of 1990 (OFPA) is overseen by the federal government for standards set regarding the production, processing and certification of **organic** food in the United States.

In addition, The National Organic Standards Board

was established to develop both specific guidelines and procedures to federally regulate all **organic** crops in the U.S.

Since the USDA's implementation of the NOP in October 2002, all food labeled "**organic**" must meet the aforementioned national organic standards.

It should be clarified that while most distributors work hard to earn their USDA "**organic**" seal of approval, the use of the seal IS voluntary. Just remember in order to wear the "**organic**" badge, products must contain 95% or more NOP regulated **organic** ingredients.

The penalty for using a USDA organic label or selling food products with a USDA **organic** label without meeting USDA certified **organic** standards carries a $10,000 fine per violation.

Organic Vs. Non-Organic

What are the benefits to buying **organic** food?

First of all, (and for some, most importantly) there is the taste. The argument can be made that better-tasting, pesticide-free fresh produce will encourage more people to follow mom's advice to eat their fruits and veggies. Also there's the assumption that because organic produce, specifically, tastes better that you may buy less. Quality over quantity.

"There is definitely a difference in flavor and texture of an organic product," said Perry McNeese, general manager at Good Earth Market, which specializes in organic and locally produced items.

But are **organic** foods actually better for you?

The American Journal of Clinical Nutrition recently reported from over 50 research studies that there is no solid evidence that organic food carries higher nutritional content than its' non-organic counterparts.

"It wasn't brand-new news," said Lindsey Diemert, a registered dietician and licensed nutritionist at Billings Clinic.

However, the option for pesticide-free produce can hardly be a bad one. Lowering the risk of chemical-ridden food and minimizing their intake is well worth going **organic** for most people who choose to "go green". Which leads us to the next question...

Is Organic Food Safer?

In that **organic** food contains no pesticides, antibiotics, or genetically modified ingredients, the short answer to that is: YES.

Experts agree that even small doses of pesticide residue in conventionally grown foods are potentially harmful to humans, particularly unborn babies and children. Pesticides in food have been linked to a host of health-risk diseases including cancer, alzheimer's, obesity, and birth defects in unborn babies.

For a complete list of pesticides found in common supermarket produce refer to this <u>Organic</u>

Produce Pesticide Chart at: http://www.bellybytes.com/articles/organic-produce-table.html

As for the hazardous health effects of eating hormone-laden and genetically-modified foods, there may not be sufficient signifiers yet linked, but common sense says minimizing intake is a smart idea. Industrial livestock farms routinely administer antibiotics are to farm animals to enhance growth or prevent disease. Having scientific evidence that overuse of antibiotics leads to resistant certain helpful strains of bacteria in the human body, makes antibiotic-injected food sources a grave concern for consumers.

In general, the USDA has been very clear, however, to go on the record as saying that the **organic** seal is a confirmation of a specific method of production and not a federally approved stamp of approval as a safety endorsement.

"Go Green" for the Environment

Organic agriculture considers the long-term effect of

agricultural interventions on the ecosystem. It aims to produce food while establishing an ecological balance in maximizing soil fertility without the total elimination of pesky pest problems. **Organic** farming takes a proactive approach, looking at the longterm benefit, as opposed to treating problems after they emerge.

Organic farming also reduces the length of time that soil is exposed to erosive forces is decreased, so soil biodiversity is encouraged, thereby reducing nutrient loss, helping to maintain and enhance soil productivity.

Ideally, **organic** farming uses less energy. It also minimizes pollution of air and groundwater and helps maintain long-term soil fertility.

In many agriculture areas, pollution of groundwater is caused by synthetic fertilizers and pesticides, which is obviously a major problem. As the use of these are prohibited in **organic** farming, they are replaced by things like ompost, animal manure, and green manure enhancing soil structure while keeping neighboring waterways pure.

The use of GMOs is strictly prohibited in any stage of **organic** food production, processing, or handling. As the potential impact of GMOs to both the environment and health is not entirely understood, **organic** agriculture takes a precautionary approach to GMO-related risk factors by choosing to encourage natural biodiversity.

By buying organic, the consumer through his/her purchasing power promotes a less polluting agricultural system. The hidden cost of agro-agriculture (paid for in our taxes) to the environment in terms of natural resource degradation is reduced.

Top Reasons People Are Opting Organic[4]

To avoid pesticides: 70.3%

Freshness: 68.3%

Health and nutrition: 67.1%

Prevention of genetically modified foods: 55 percent%

How to Switch to Organic Foods

Here are some practical steps to make the switch to Go Green:

Resist the urge to buy **organic** everything all at once, Even switching to a few **organic** selections on a regular basis makes a difference.

Start by making the switch to **organic** versions of everyday mainstays. Try **organic** milk, cheese, pasta, and produce.

Try different brands of **organic** options every time you shop. Also try new and different **organic** options altogether like organic tofu, stuffed vine leaves, and soup. EXPERIMENT!

Try shopping for your **organic** foods at local farmers markets and support your **organic**community!

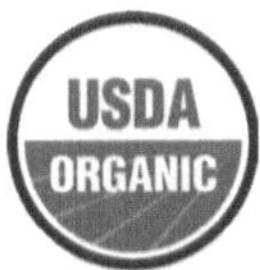

Organic foods will become less expensive as the demand for them increase... Shop **Organic** & Shop Wisely!

We pay through our taxes for the hidden (absorbed) costs of cleaning up our polluted waterways from chemical runoff of mass-produced agro-agriculture.

Once you've gone green, you'll quickly appreciate the many advantages of eating **organic** foods... And you won't ever switch back.

Which organic foods should I buy?

Many experts recommend eating **organic** meats, dairy, and eggs when possible, though as previously mentioned this can be challenging, given non-GMO standards. Store-bought **organic** baby food is a good idea, or better yet, make your own from **organic** food ingredients.

For produce, it's wise to buy **organic** for the "dirty dozen." These twelve fruits and veggies contained the most pesticide residues when tested by the not-for-profit Environmental Working Group. They are:

Peaches

Apples

Sweet Bell Peppers

Celery

Nectarines

Strawberries

Cherries

Pears

Grapes (Imported)

Spinach

Lettuce

Potatoes

For a printable, pocket-sized shopper's guide to pesticides in produce, visit www.foodnews.org

Why is Organic Food so Expensive?

Organic products typically cost 10-40% more than similar conventionally produced products. Certified **organic** products are generally more expensive than conventional counterparts for a number of reasons:

Organic food supply is limited as compared to demand; Production for organic food typically costs more because of increased labor cost.

Marketing and the distribution for **organic** products is relatively inefficient as small quantities of food are being shipped.

As the demand for **organic** food products increases, technological innovations will reduce costs of production, processing, and distribution of **organic** produce. It's also a matter of simple economics…The greater the demand, the lower the price of produce. Vote with your dollars! Go Green with your green!

10 Tips for Eating Organic on a Budget

1) BUY LOCAL! Buy fresh produce from your local farmer's market. Fresh produce from the supermarket is more expensive and not as fresh, even if it's marked **organic**. Skip the middlemen and lower your expense.

2) If you have a local Co-op Distributor, join it. Co-ops operate for the benefit of their members and are usually able to offer services and products at lower prices, with less market price markup.

For a list of Co-op Distributors, visit: http://
www.coopdirectory.org/distributor.htm

3) Stick to the basics. Start with the "dirty dozen" list of **organic** produce "must-have"s and go from there.

4) Eat every part of your fruits and veggies… Don't waste the stems and skins!

5) Make a shopping list that doesn't include convenience foods, which are often more costly than fresh raw ingredients you can buy and store.

6) Try eating less meat by making dishes with alternative high-protein ingredients like lentils and beans.

7) Grow your own **organic** garden! Even if it's just a window box of fresh herbs in a or a pot of juicy tomatoes.

8) For certain types of foods, especially the dry varieties which will keep for longer periods, try buying in bulk.

9) Bake your own bread and baked goods. Try a bread machine if you're feeling lazy.

10) Forage for wild food on hikes. You can find everything from fresh herbs to just-ripened fruit if you look carefully.

Still thirsty for more? There is a plethora of information out there on the history and progression of Organic farming, as well as Resources for those choosing an Organic lifestyle. I'm listing some of the Organic "Best Finds" Resources below. Online sites like the ones listed are known to have links galore to similar sites, invested in Organic living. Here's a sampling to get you started.

Resources for "Going Green"

Books on Organic Living

Organic, Inc. by Samuel Fromartz

Contains a wealth of information on the history of the organics "movement", organic farming, and organic products.

A Field Guide to Buying Organic by Luddene Perry and Dan Schultz

An aisle-by-aisle supermarket guide to information about not only organic produce, dairy, meat and poultry, but also baked goods, nuts, seeds, grains, and beverages.

Organic Cookbook: Making the Most of Fresh and Seasonal Produce; 150 Deliciously Healthy Recipes Shown in 250 Stunning Photographs by YsanneSpevack Having scripted over a dozen cookbooks and an organic advocate tour de force, this is the first of a series of cookbooks filled with delicious organic recipes.

Online Resources

Organic Consumers Association's GreenPeople Directory: http://www.organicconsumers.org/btc/BuyingGuide.cfm

The Organic Center: http://www.organic-center.org/res.consumer.html

The Organic Trade Association: http://www. howtogoorganic.com/

Movement Exercises

Machines vs. Free Weights and Bodyweight

People often say that they use machines because they are safer and convenient. Basically, people like machines because they are easier. Machines require you to push or pull on a guided path, with no balance, coordination, or proprioception needed. More importantly, the body's nervous system is "wired" to work in sections, therefore negating the positive effects of working as a system of multiple muscles. This considerably slows progress.

We already know from the material in this book that the more intensity used, the more we can take advantage of EPOC. The effects of EPOC will last longer by including free weights and bodyweight exercises in your workouts. Bodyweight and free weight training add the intensity needed to achieve maximum fat loss. Overall, free weights and bodyweight exercises will outperform machine training in terms of conditioning and fat loss every time. Sitting in a machine won't get you the muscle involvement that you get by lifting weights. Several machines are needed to match the effectiveness of exercises like the clean and jerk and the snatch. To achieve the ultimate in fat loss, train using free weights and your bodyweight.

Warm-Up/Cool Down

The warm-up is an often forgotten aspect of training programs. I know you're ready to work out—you finally have the motivation to get to the gym or have made the time to work out at your home gym—and the last thing you want is another hold up to starting your workout. Or, maybe you're running late to your workout and decide to skip the warm-up altogether. This is not a good decision. The warm-up helps protect you from injuries that hamper your results and aids in ensuring that your workouts are productive and efficient. Warm-ups serve to raise body temperature, increase blood flow to the muscles, and notify the body that there will be activity. The warm-up also stimulates the nervous system, which elevates coordination and balance.

There are several different ways to warm up: static, general, and specific. Trying to figure out the best way to prepare your muscles for the training session can be a very confusing task.

Let's start with static stretches. By their very name, these stretches are based on lack of movement. Lack of movement is the opposite of fitness training, not to mention sports training. Slow movements, as well as multi-direction and maximum effort movements, are a part of fitness programs; therefore, using movement-based warm-ups for fitness and sports activities is only logical. I believe that static stretching has a place in your training but they should not be done before your workouts. I recommend that you do static stretching after your workouts, to recover and relax.

Next, a general warm-up increases heart and respiratory rates, and blood flow, which delivers oxygen and nutrients to working muscles. All of this aids in preparing muscles, tendons, and joints for activity. Perform your general warm-up for ten to fifteen minutes and spend a couple of minutes on each exercise.

Finally, specific warm-ups involve the exact movements or exercises that will occur in the workout. Specific warm-ups are the most accurate activities because they prepare the nervous system with the exact blueprint for what will transpire when you escalate the movements to full speed. Perform your first round of workouts at 50% effort, followed by rounds at 70% and 85%. When your body feels warm, start your workout at 100% effort.

There are many different thoughts on proper warm-ups. For this reason, I have listed three different warm-up modalities to choose from. Use the warm-up method that you are most comfortable with, but please don't skip the warm-up. It's an essential part of your workout for performance reasons and will help guard against injury.

General Warm-Up

The following general warm-up exercises increase heart and respiratory rates, and blood flow, and help prepare muscles, tendons, and joints for activity. As noted earlier, perform your general warm-up for ten to fifteen minutes and spend a couple of minutes on each exercise.

Jump Rope

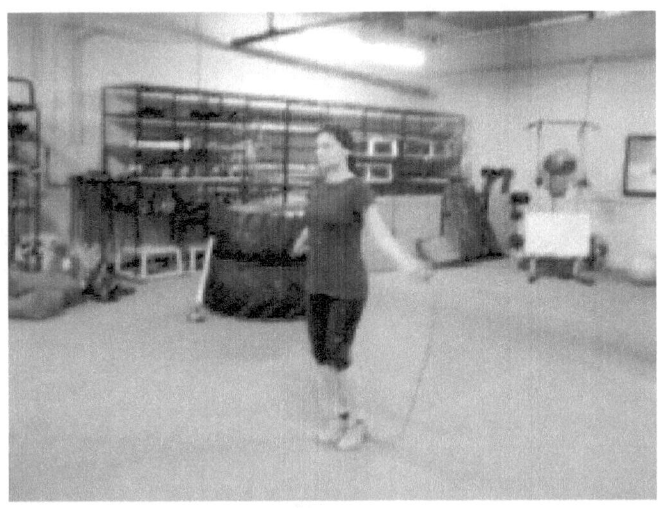

Swing the rope over your head in a forward motion, keeping your feet together while jumping over the rope. You may increase your speed and reps as you feel more comfortable.

Iron Cross

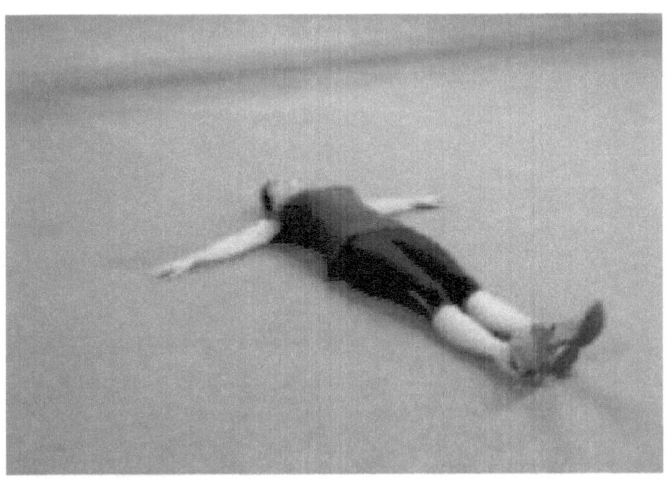

Lay flat on your back with your arms out to your sides. Bring your right leg over and try to have it touch your left hand. Switch and bring your left leg over and touch it with your left hand. Try to keep your back flat on the ground.

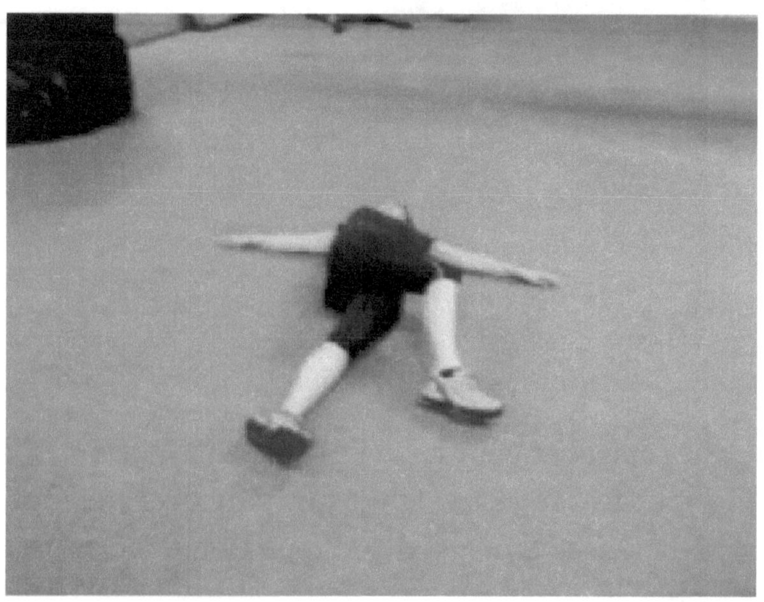

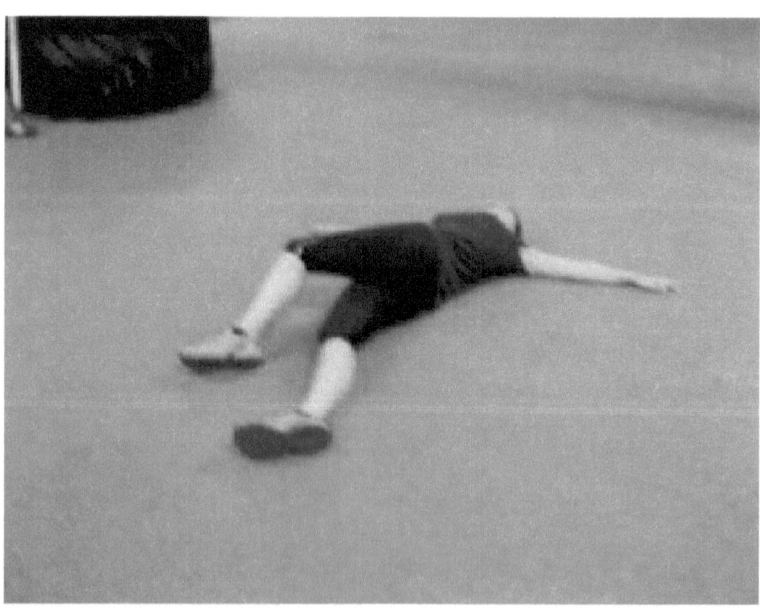

Lateral Steps

A cardio movement, definitely not a long, slow cardio exercise. Perform the exercise by moving side-to-side and repeating the motion.

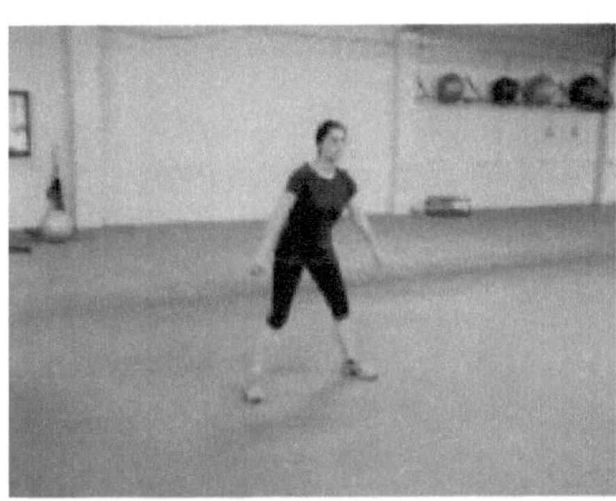 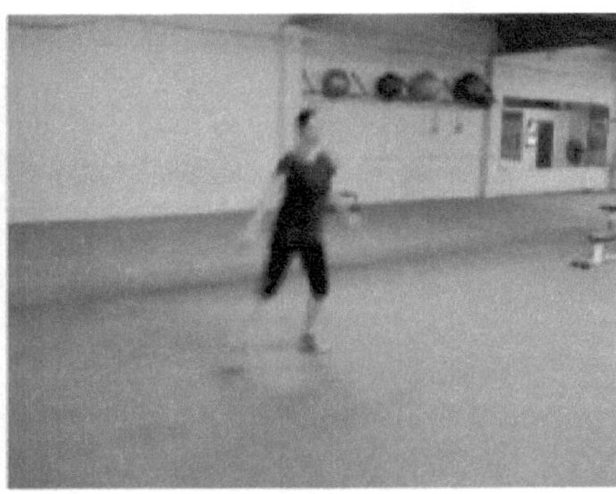

Run in Place

Run in place for 20-second intervals.

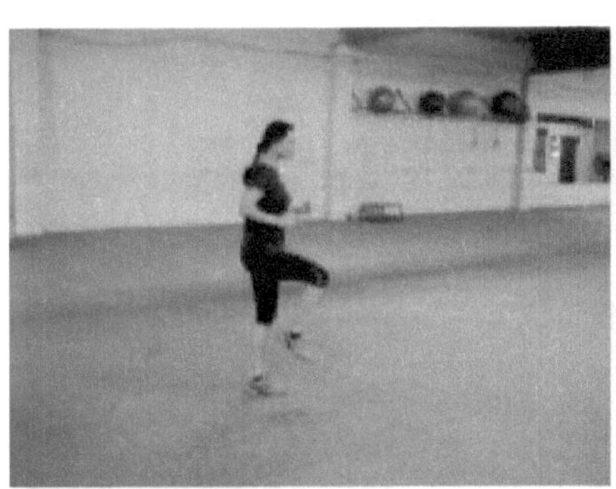 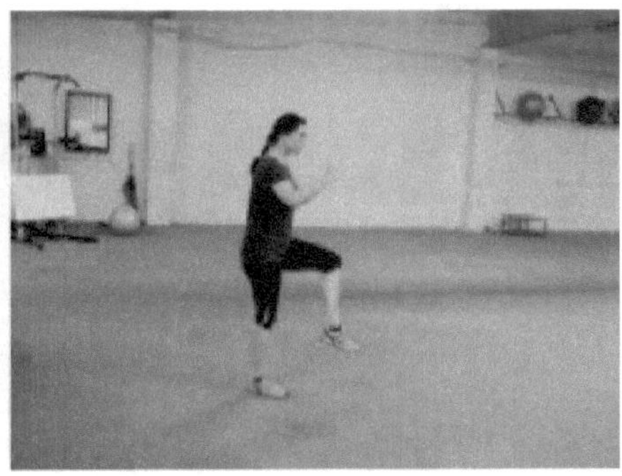

Alternate Hamstring Stretch

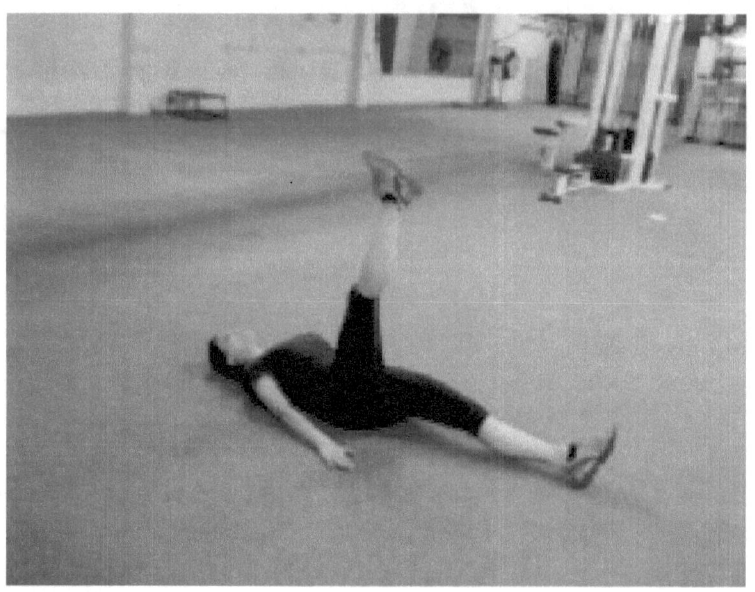

To begin, lay flat on your back with your arms out to your sides. Bring one leg up as far as you can. Alternate legs.

Jumping Jacks

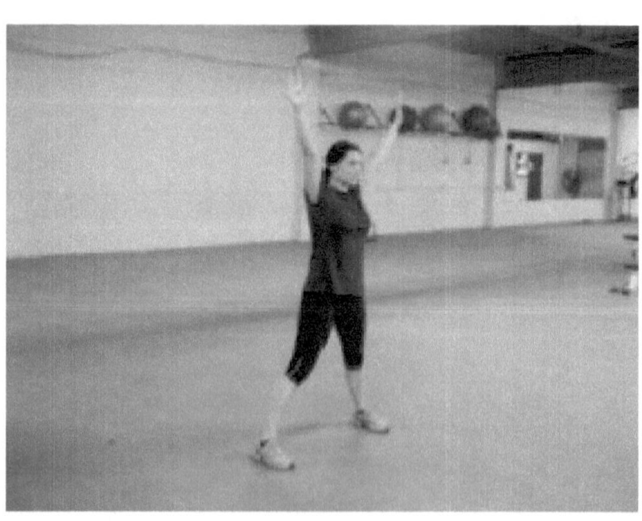

Start with hands and feet together. Jump your feet to the sides, at the same time bring your arms above your head and return to the starting position. Repeat the movement.

Skipping

Start by bringing your leg up in the air as the opposite arm swings forward. Continue for 20 to 30 yards. Always keep your chest up.

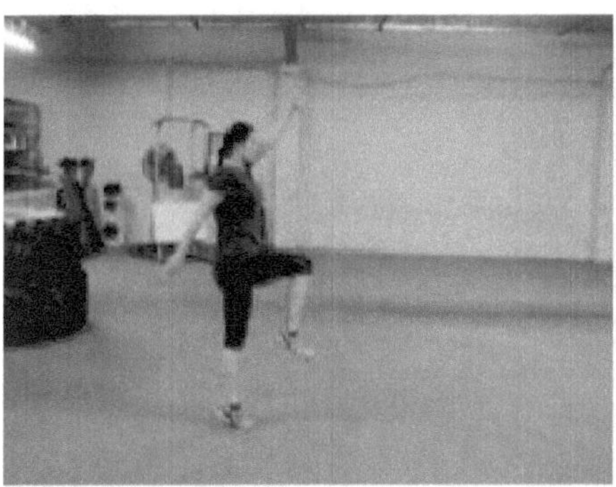 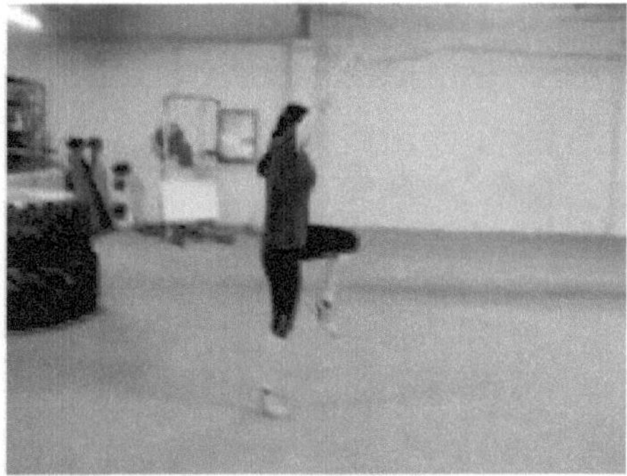

Cross Overs

Stand in a lateral position and bring one leg across the other leg. Continue for 20 to 30 yards by switching legs, one over the other. Keep your chest up and your shoulders back.

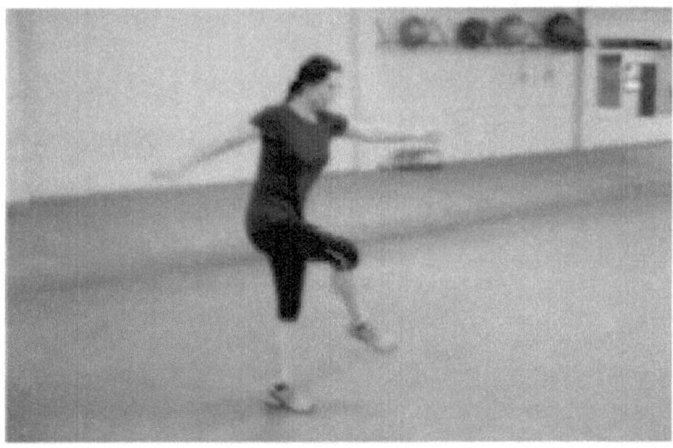

Static Stretches

As we discussed earlier, static stretches are based on lack of movement. Static stretching has its place in your training but not before your workouts. Do the following static stretches after your workouts, to recover and relax.

Back Stretch

Lie with your back on the ground. With your arms, pull your knees to your chest and hold the stretch for approximately 25 to 30 seconds.

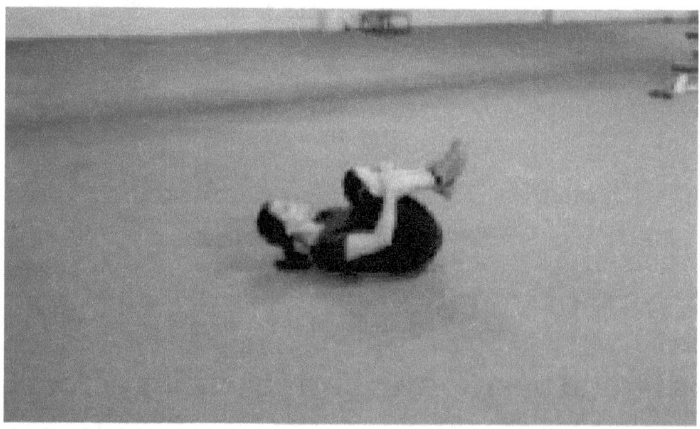

Buddha Stretch

Sit on the floor and use your elbows to press your knees apart. Hold the position while keeping your chest up in a good postural position. Hold for 25 to 30 seconds.

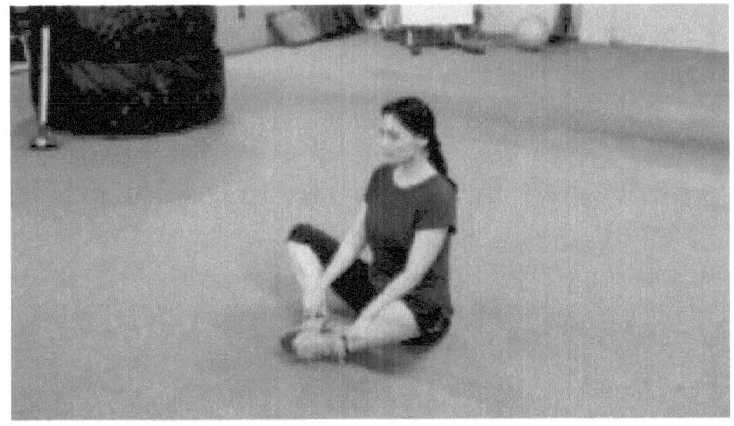

Cat Stretch

Place yourself on your hands and knees on the floor. Suck your belly button towards your spine and tuck your chin towards your chest. Curl your back like a cat and hold the position for 25 to 30 seconds.

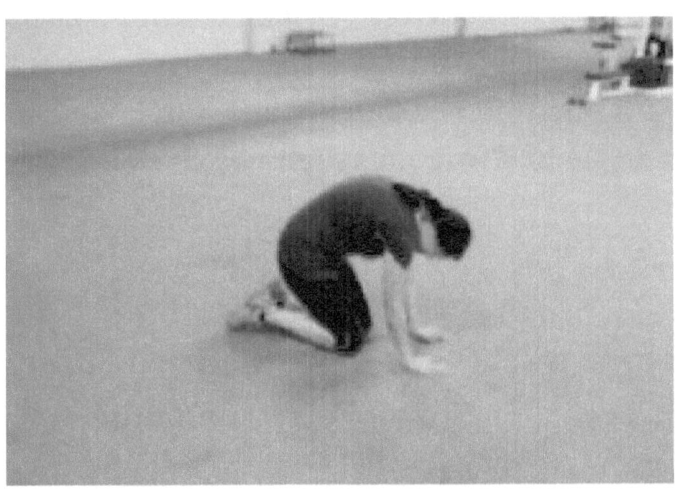

Hip Stretch

Lie flat on the floor with your arms stretched out. Anchor your upper body to the floor and your lower body goes to one side with both knees facing the same side. Hold stretch for 25 to 30 seconds.

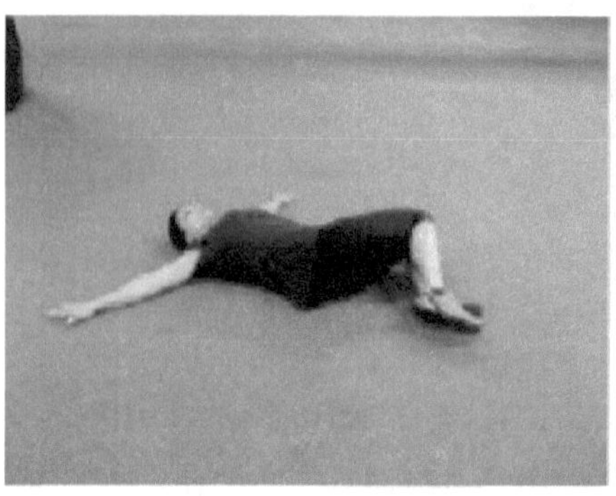 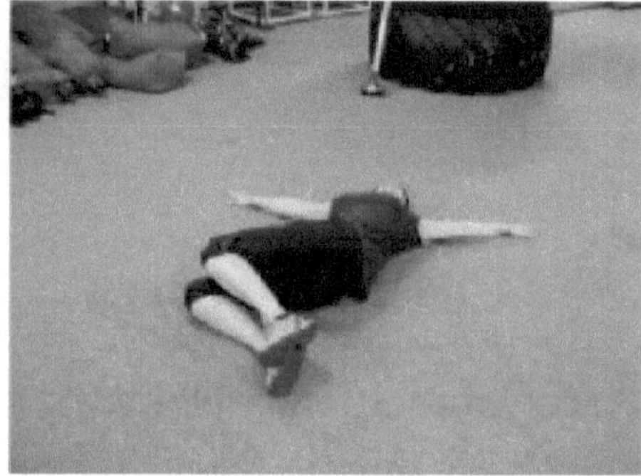

Hurdle Stretch

Sit flat on the floor, bend one leg, and face the sole of that foot to the other leg. Point your toes in the air and reach out to pull your outstretched foot toward your body. Hold the position for 25 to 30 seconds then switch sides.

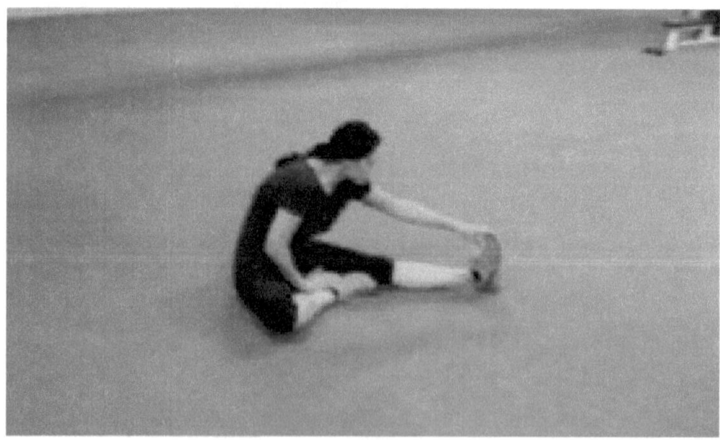

Pretzel Stretch

Sit on the floor and cross one leg over the other. Turn and look to the opposing side and push against that leg. Hold the position for 25 to 30 seconds then switch sides.

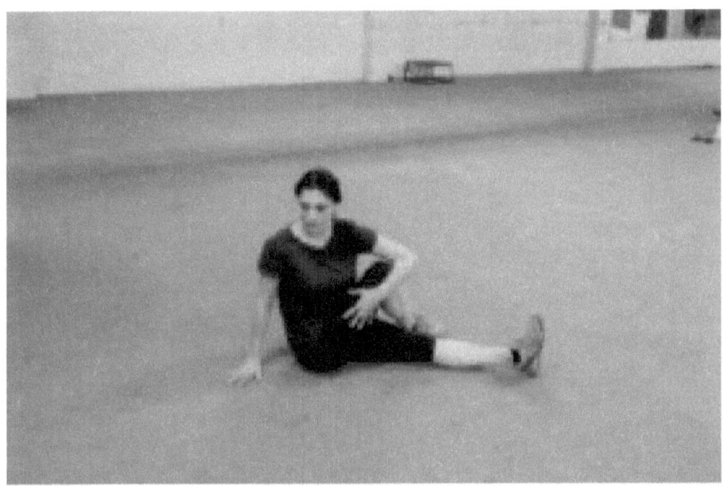

Quad Stretch

Stand straight up and grab your ankle, pulling it upwards, toward the ceiling. Look straight up and keep your chest up. Hold the position for 25 to 30 seconds then switch sides.

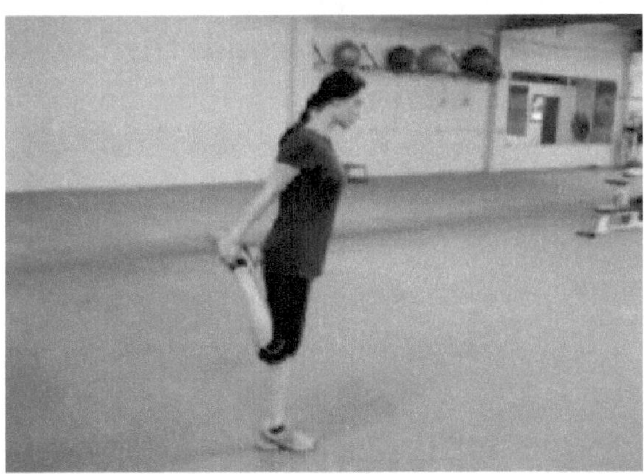

Deltoid Stretch

Stand straight up and pull one arm across your body to feel a stretch throughout your shoulder area and into your upper back. Hold the position for 25 to 30 seconds then

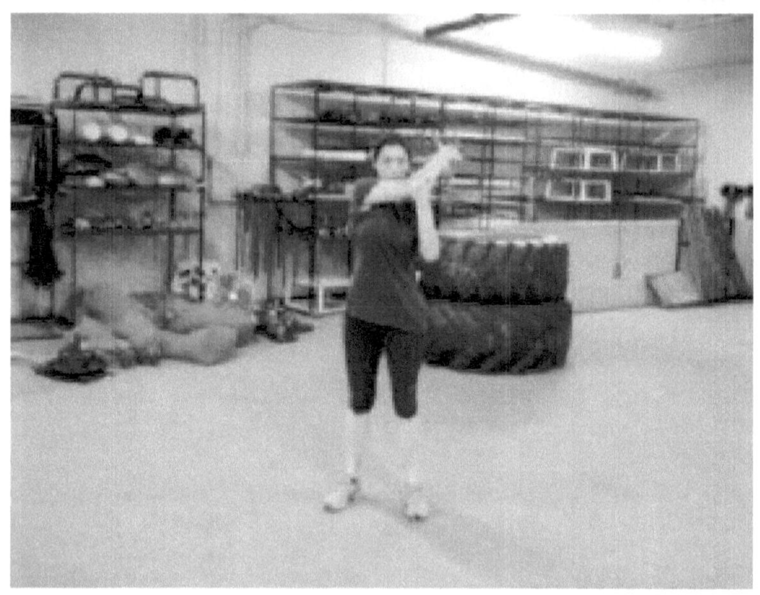

Chest Stretch

Stand with your lower arm braced against a pole. Turn your body slightly away from the pole until you feel a stretch. Hold the position for 25 to 30 seconds then switch sides.

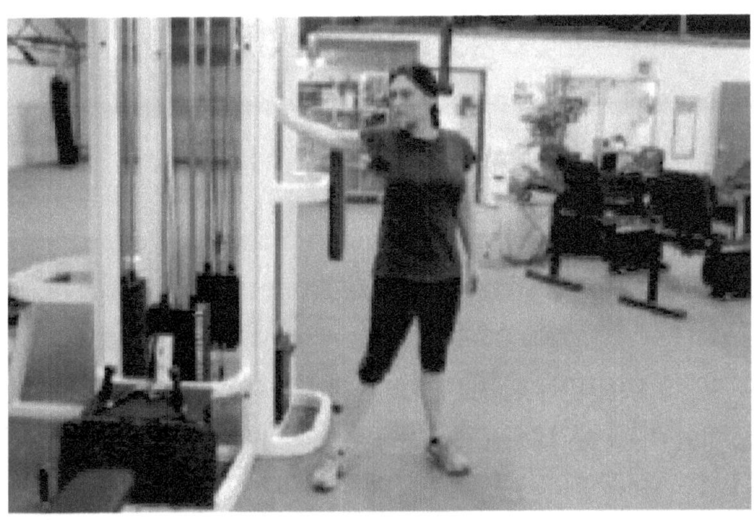

Abdominal Stretch

Anchor your lower body into the ground then raise your upper body off the ground. This will insure a stretch in the abdominal area. Hold the position for 25 to 30 seconds.

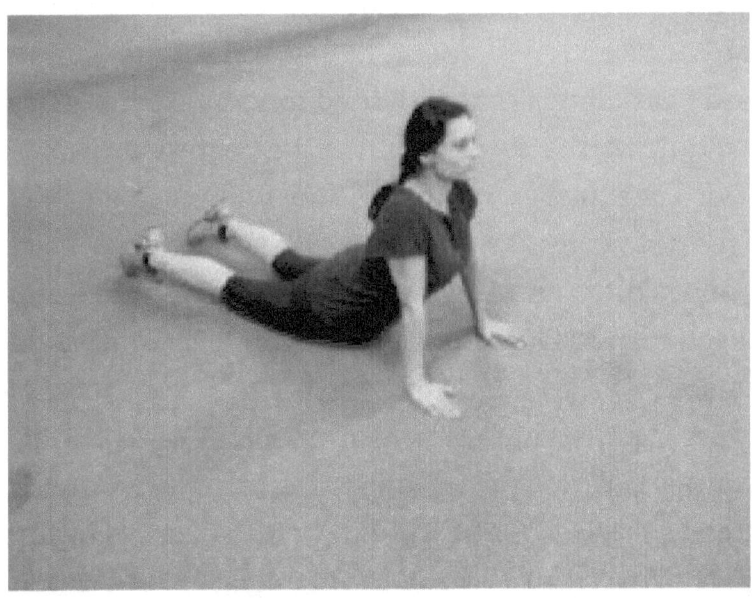

Program Design

In this section, I describe seventy-one fat-burning, muscle-building exercises, and variations that you can choose from. I have also split the exercises into three groups: beginning, intermediate, and advanced.

After this section, I will give you five different workout combinations for each level, and all can be mixed and matched. Remember that no workout is right or wrong. I also provide you with starting points from which you may design your workouts to suit your body and your individual needs.

The exercises in the beginner group are basic but still challenging. We all know how difficult squats and deadlifts can be, but they are still called basic exercises. Difficulty in an exercise comes in two ways, the first comes by adding load while doing the exercise and the second is by adding forward or lateral movement, i.e., lateral squats or side and forward bear crawls may be added to increase intensity.

Train twice a week while in the beginner's group. Start with the first workout and stay with each workout for three or four weeks, then move to the next workout. Everyone is different. If you think you need more time, stay with each respective workout until you feel comfortable moving on. Remember, adjust routines to your fitness level

Essentially, the training protocol for each group determines the group's difficulty. Yes, there are some advanced exercises that I wouldn't put in the beginning group. However, once you've spent at least four weeks in each group, all exercises may be mixed and matched using the protocols provided, or by using workouts that you have created to add variety and to suit your personal goals.

Deadlift

Step up to the barbell with your feet approximately shoulder width apart. The bar should be close to your shins and over the balls of your feet. Squat down and grab the bar with a grip slightly wider than shoulder width. Lower your thighs until they are parallel to the floor. Keep your chest up and look straight ahead. Initiate the movement by pushing through the ground to extend your hips and straighten your legs. Keep your arms straight throughout the entire movement. Come to a standing position, with straight posture and with shoulders back. The bar will be resting on your hips as you stand straight. Lower the bar by initiating with the hips, bending the knees, and keeping the chest up.

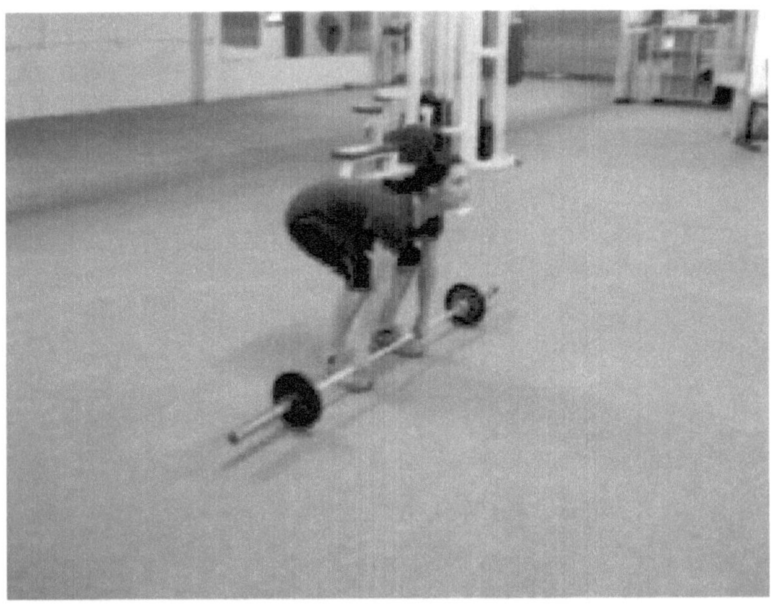

Dumbbell Deadlift

Lower yourself in a controlled manner and then stand up with the dumbbells, squeezing your glutes forward.

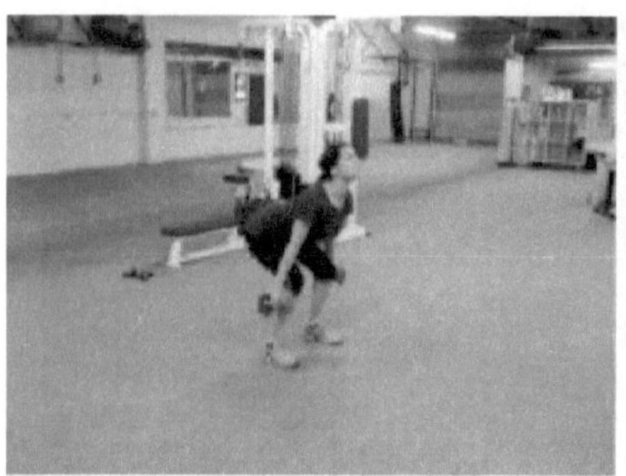
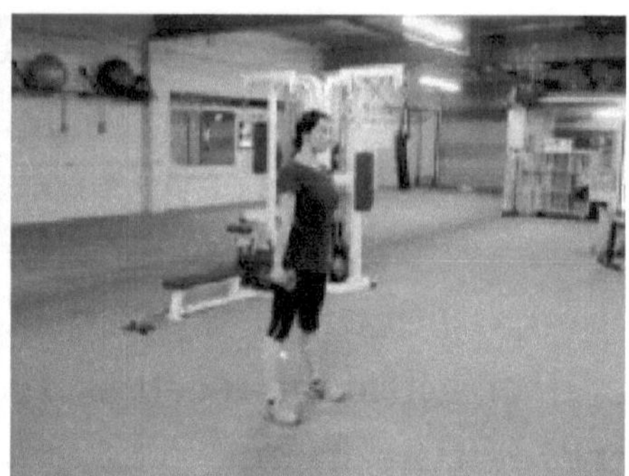

One Legged Dumbbell Deadlift

This exercise is done unilaterally, meaning one leg at a time. Your right hand will go to your left foot, and your left hand will go to your right foot. Keep your chest up and reach with the dumbbell to your shoestrings, then return to the starting position.

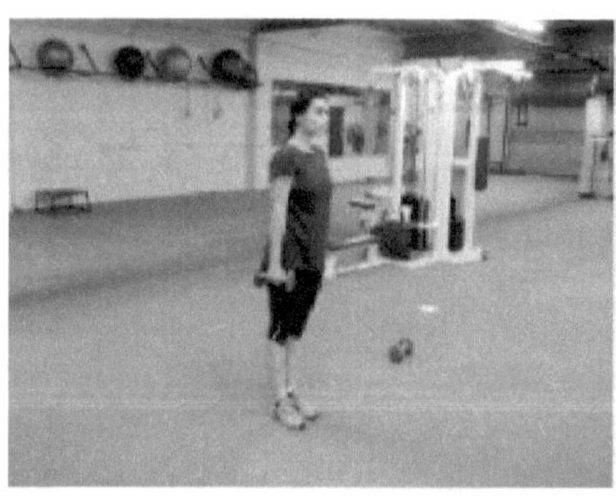
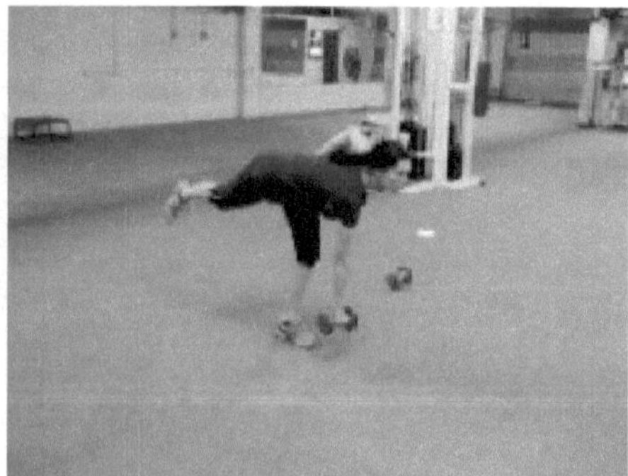

Romanian Deadlift

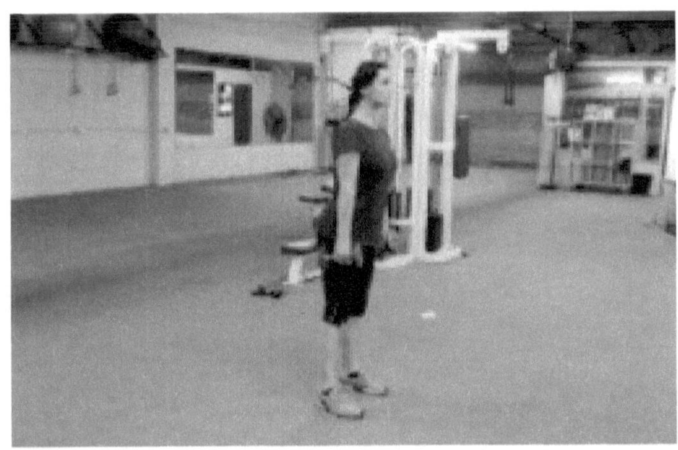

Very similar to the Good Morning but the load (weight) hangs in front of you, whereas with the Good Morning, the barbell is on your back. Have your feet slightly wider than shoulder width and put the weight of your body on your heels and on the outsides of your feet. To perform the movement, initiate by bringing the hips straight back. Hold the dumbbells at arm's length, keep your chest up, and look straight ahead. As you bring your body back, squeeze your glutes forward to do so

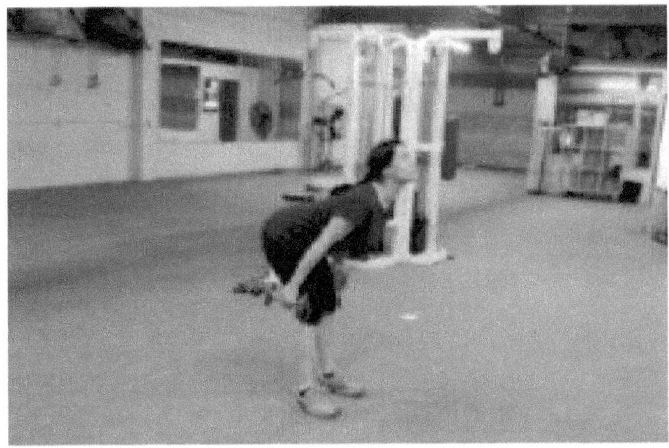

Rotational Deadlift

Grab a dumbbell with one hand and rotate to the opposite leg. Rotate the trailing leg and foot, as seen in the picture, to protect the lower back. Move to the other side and repeat. Left hand to right leg, right hand to left leg.

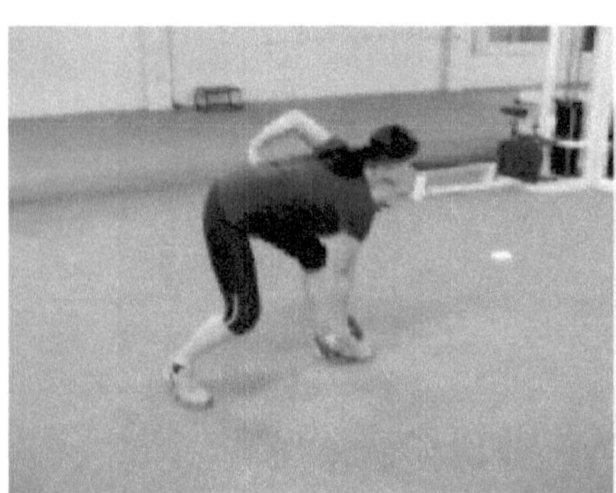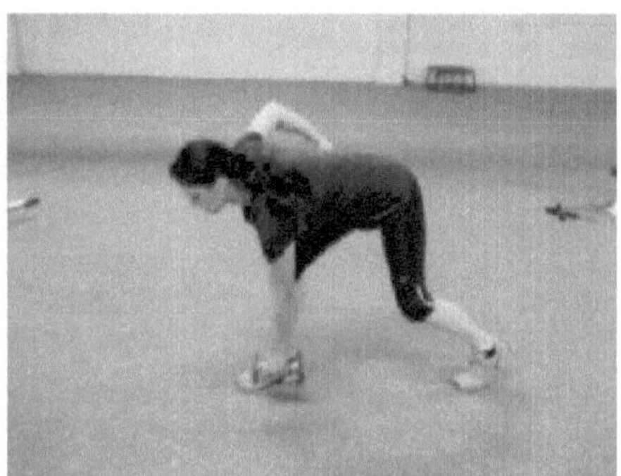

Bodyweight Squat

Position your feet shoulder width apart and your chest up while looking straight ahead. Put your bodyweight toward the heels and the outsides of your feet, to ensure that your knees stay in line with your feet and do not drift to the middle of your body. To initiate, move your hips straight back and down until they are parallel to the ground.

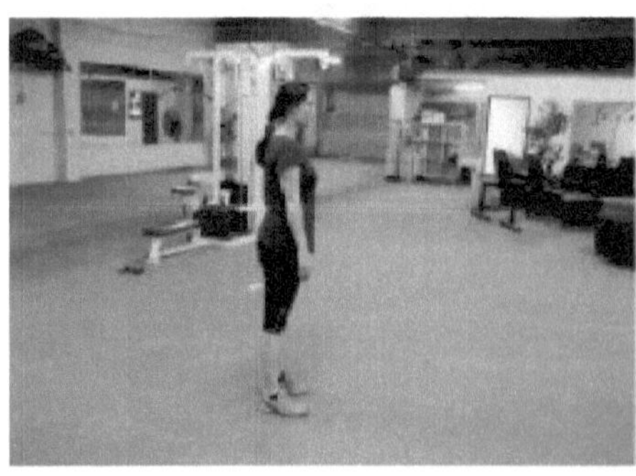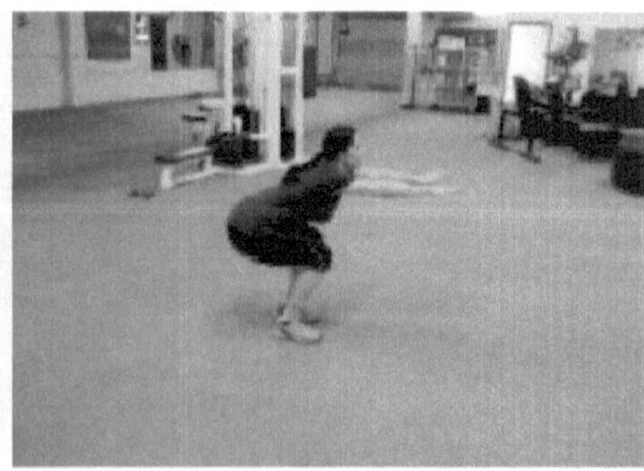

Barbell Squat

Initiate the movement by bringing the hips down and back, keeping your chest up and your eyes straight ahead. Move the weight of your body through your heels and to the outsides of your feet, to ensure that the knees stay in line with the feet and don't drift toward the midline of the body.

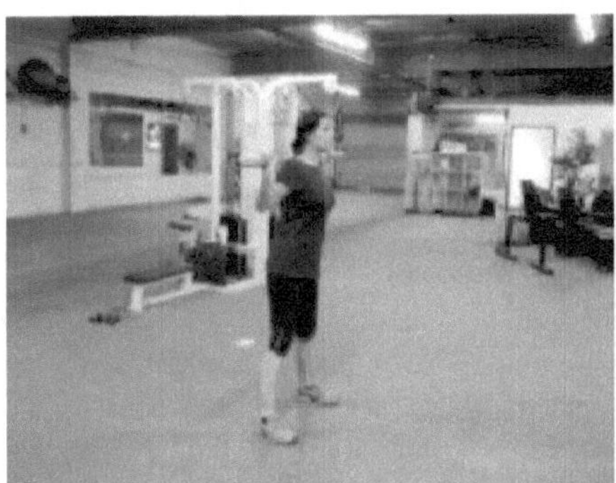
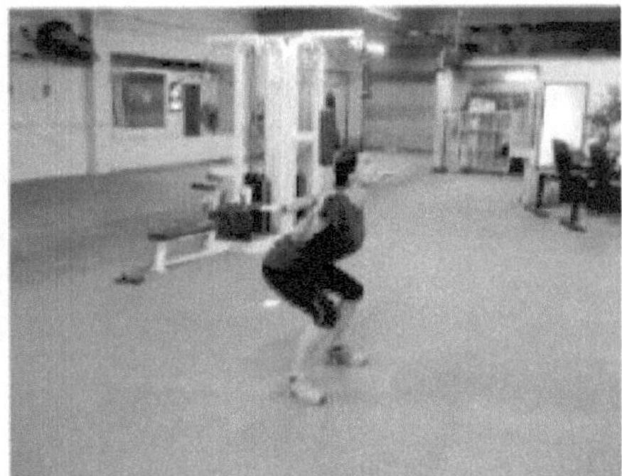

Front Squat

This is a great exercise for the quadriceps, the spinal erectors (muscles down middle of back), the abs, the hamstrings, and glutes. Lower the body to a parallel position and repeat. Keep your elbows up to hold the barbell in place.

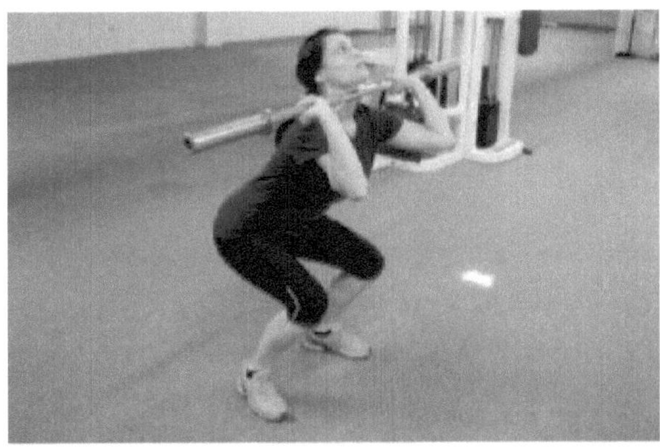

Box Squat

Start with a wide stance and initiate the movement by bringing the hips down and back to the box, then return to the starting position. This is a great movement for both beginners and advanced lifters. For the advanced lifters, the box separates the eccentric and concentric movements, making the exercise more difficult. The box serves as a landing target for beginners, therefore improving the movement.

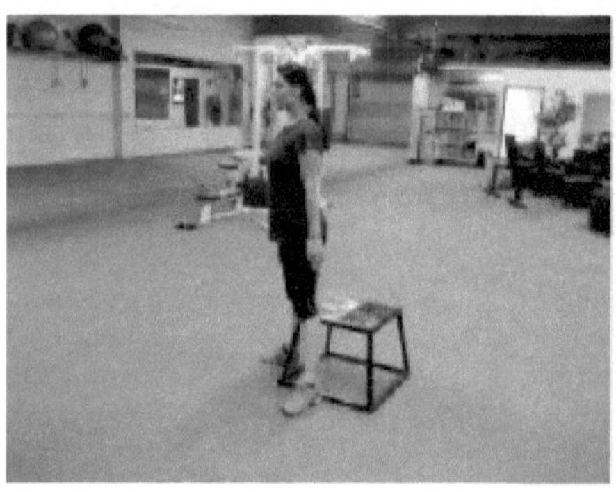 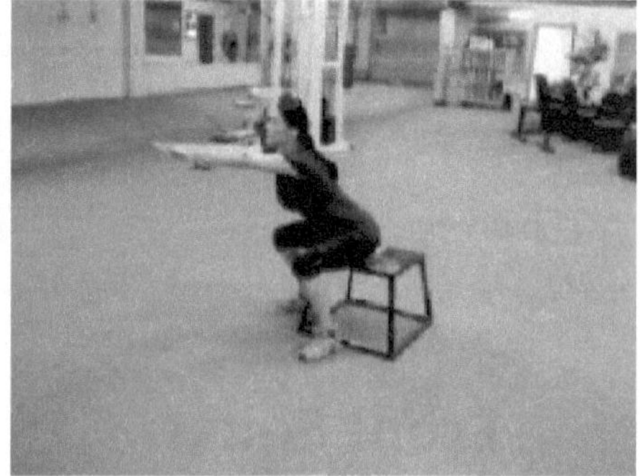

Bulgarian Squat

Start the exercise by elevating one foot on the box and keeping the other foot on the ground. Lower the back knee toward the ground, without forcing it to touch the ground, then return to the starting position. This exercise is also great for balance training.

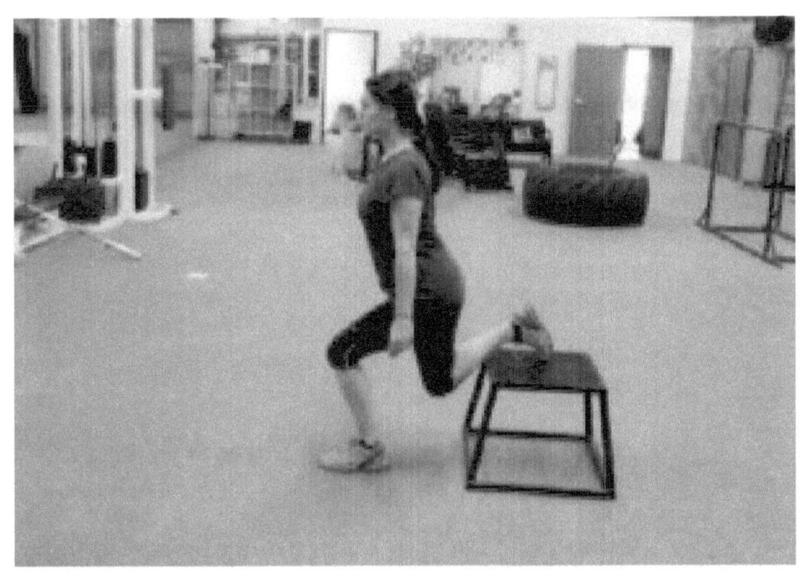

Lateral Squat

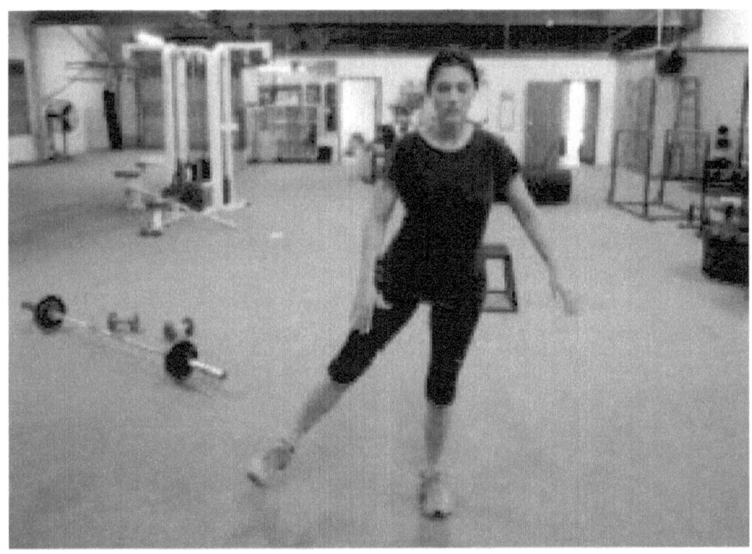

This movement, as the name implies, adds lateral
movement to the squat. Stand up straight, then as you step
to the side, lower the body like a regular squat exercise.
Keep your chest up and always look straight ahead.

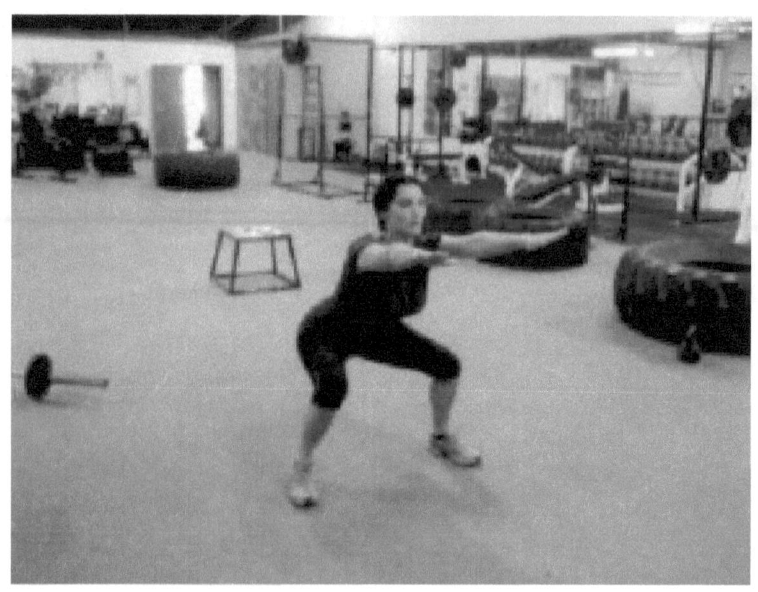

Dumbbell Overhead Squat

This is a great exercise for not only the legs but to increase flexibility through the hips and shoulder complex, and, of course, the core. Initiate the movement by bringing the hi`ps down and back while looking straight ahead and keeping your chest up. This movement also works the core to a high degree. One thing that will help is pushing through the dumbbell toward the ceiling as you're going down.

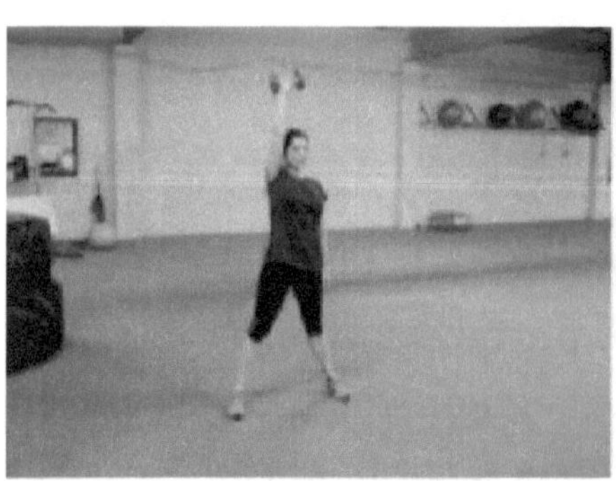

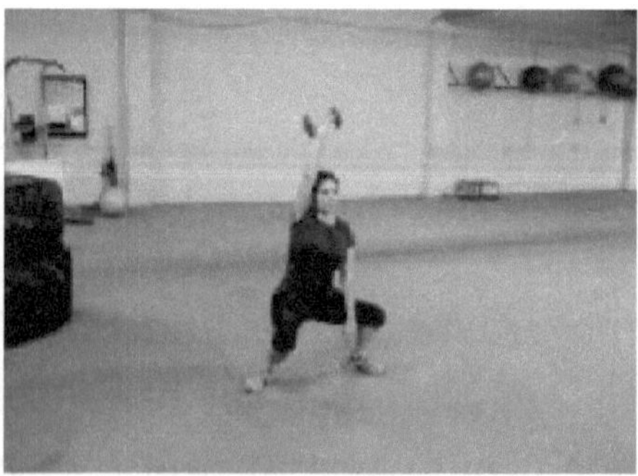

Dumbbell Squat Thrusts

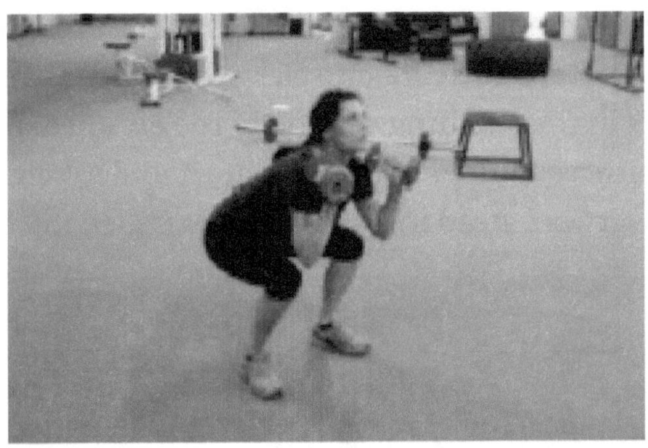

To position yourself, grab a pair of dumbbells and hold them in front of you at your shoulders. To initiate the movement, squat down with the dumbbells at shoulder level. As you come back up, press the dumbbells up smoothly, all the way to a semi-lockout, keeping your body moving in one motion. Squat down while lowering the dumbbells to your shoulders. Repeat the movement.

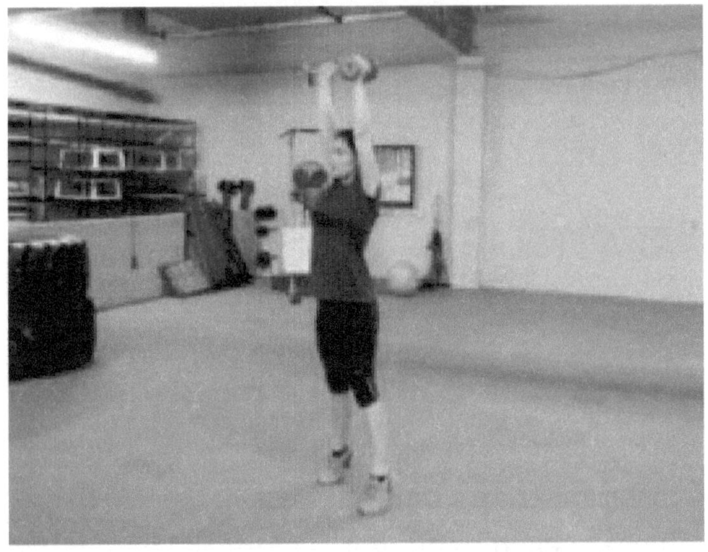

Standing Military Press

This exercise emphasizes the shoulders and also works the triceps very well. The core muscles of the upper back also play a role in the standing version of the exercise. Take the barbell with a shoulder width grip at shoulder height and press it over your head in a smooth, controlled motion.

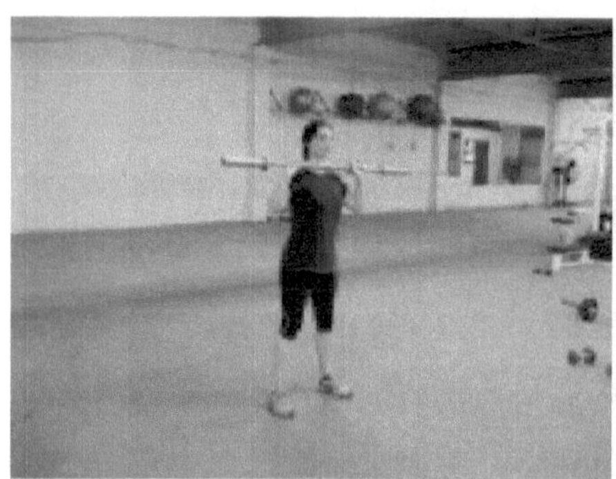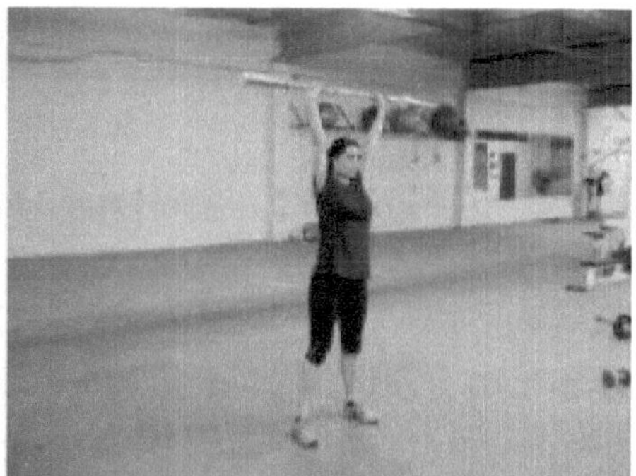

Alternate Dumbbell Chest Press

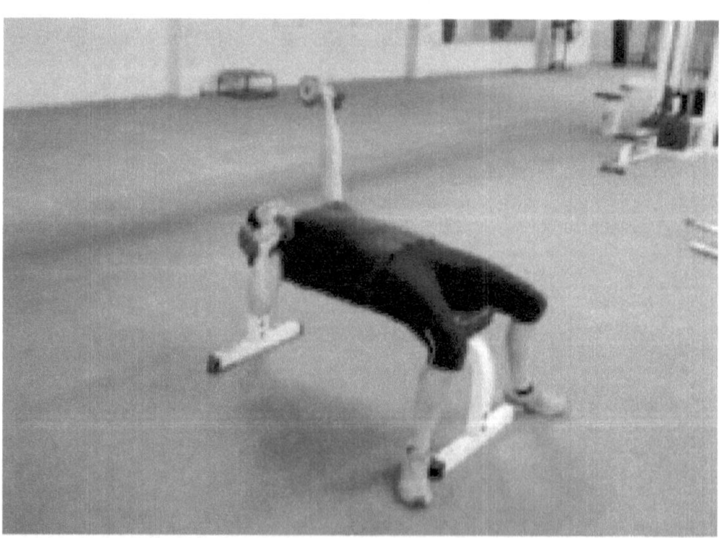

Slightly different than a barbell press in that with a dumbbell press, each hand works alone. If there is a weaker hand, it is forced to act alone. Also, more stabilizing muscles are involved when each hand works alone. Move the dumbbells in an alternating fashion. Your hands can face each other or face outward. Use different hand positions to work the chest from different angles.

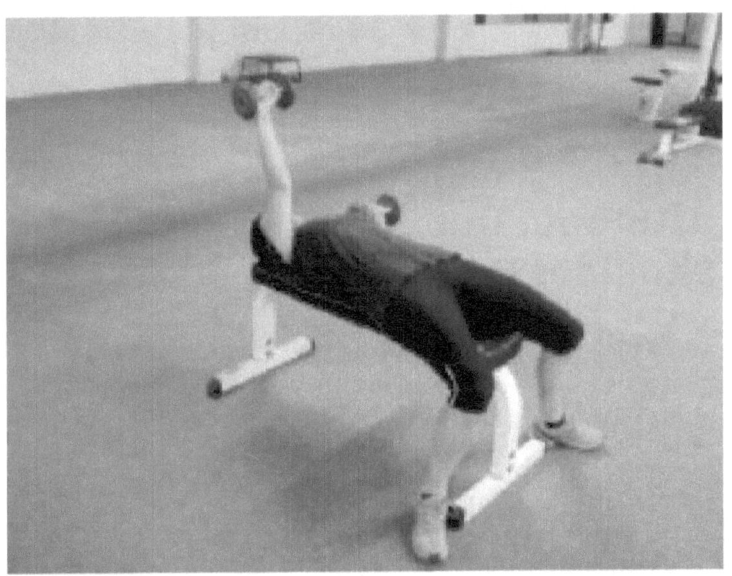

Standing Dumbbell Shoulder Press

To do the movement, press the dumbbells straight up while keeping your arms in line with your ears. You can face your palms either outward or at each other. Make sure to keep your knees bent and always look straight ahead.

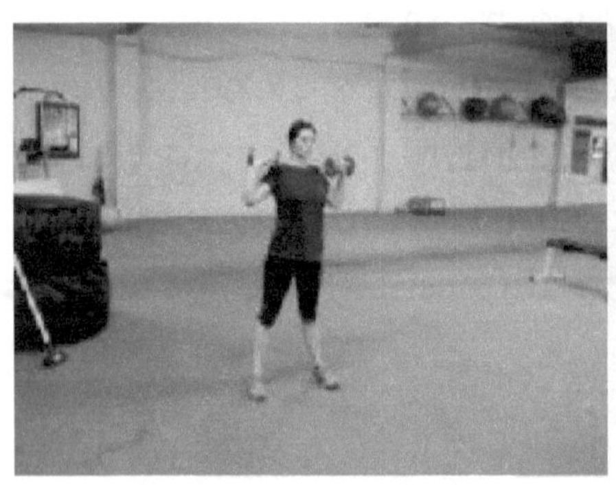 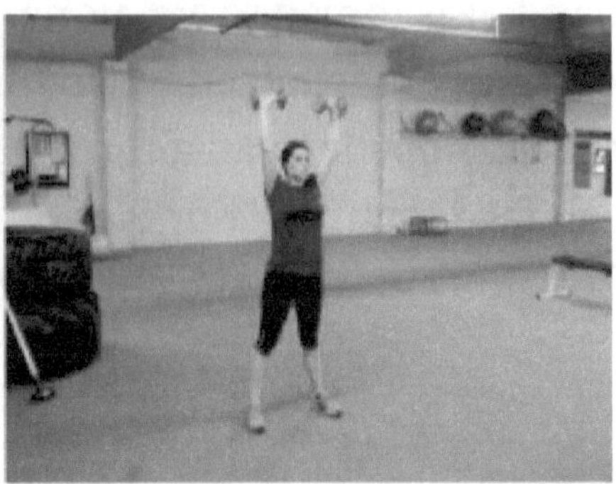

Alternate Dumbbell Standing Shoulder Press

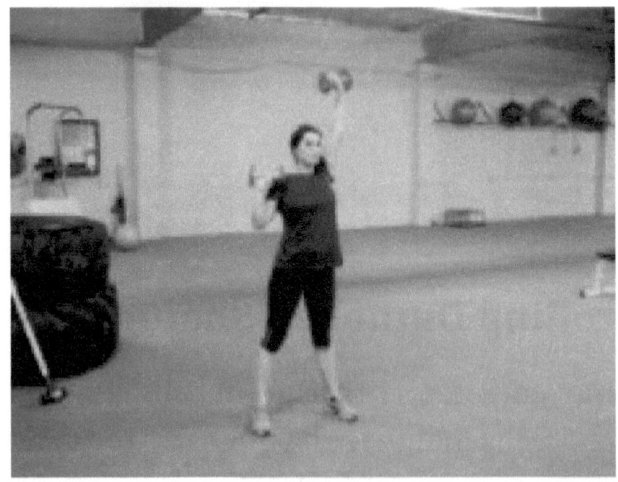

Start the movement by slightly bending the knees and keeping your chest up. Press the dumbbells up in the air, keeping the arms in line with the ears. This movement will bring in core and balance training because you are standing and not seated in a machine.

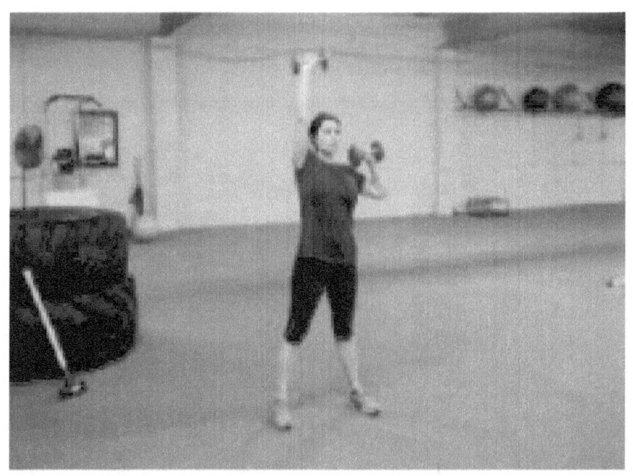

Bent Over Barbell Row

This is a great multi-joint movement exercise for the lats and the spinal erectors. Take a shoulder width stance with your glutes out and your chest up to ensure that your back stays flat.

Pull the barbell at an angle toward your belly button, with your elbows going straight back.

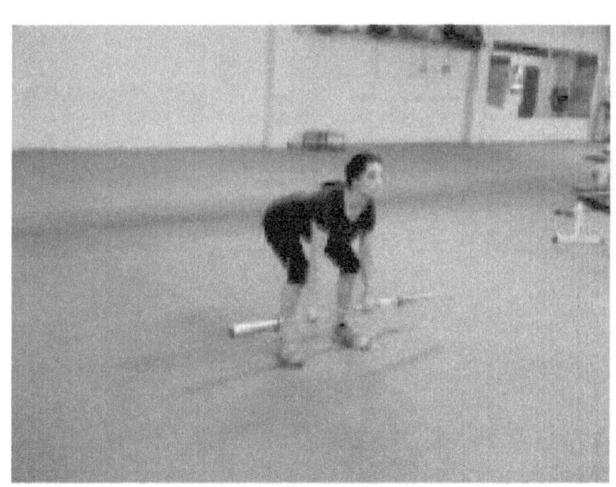 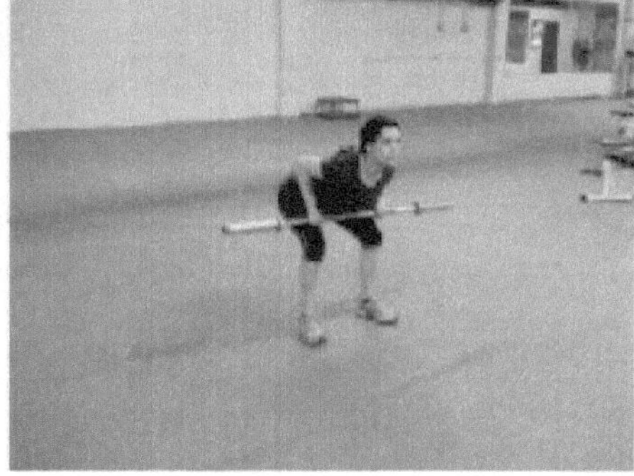

Upright Rows

Grab a pair of dumbbells and focus on pulling the elbows up then taking them down. Keep your chest up and look straight ahead.

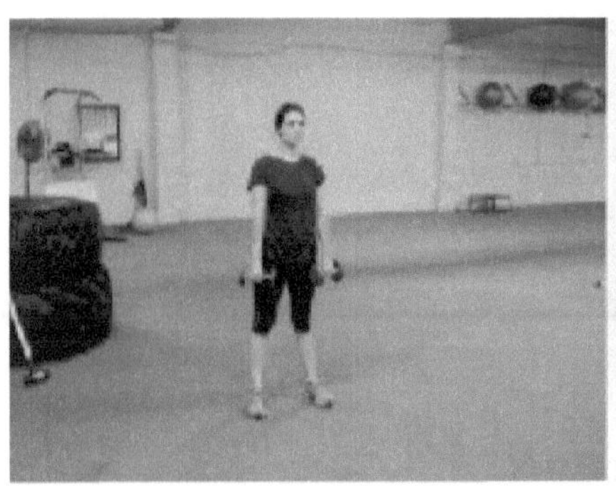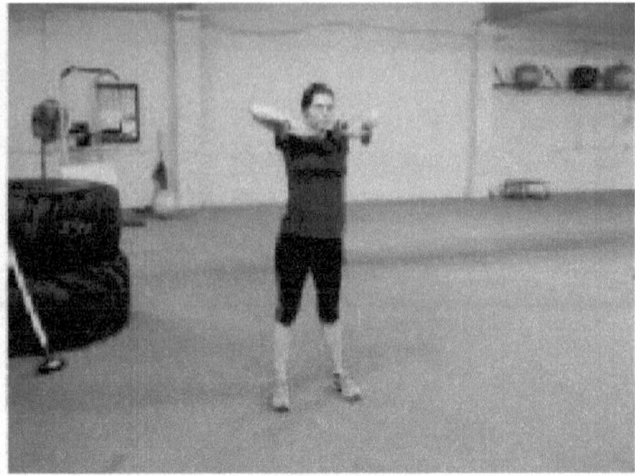

Alternate Dumbbell Rotational Rows

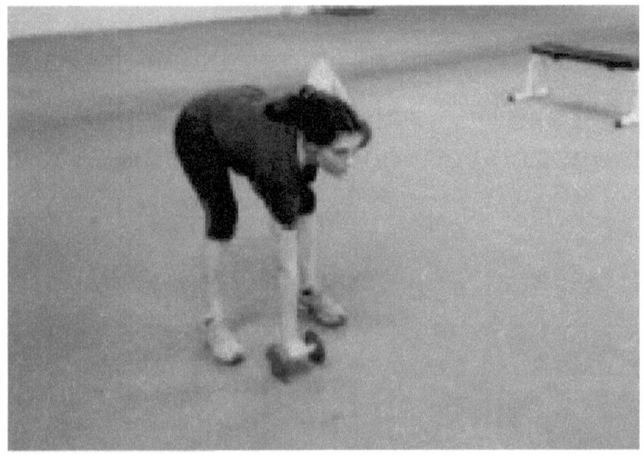

In this exercise, keep your chest up and your butt back, and your knees slightly bent. Grab a pair of dumbbells and face your palms to each other. Focus on pulling one elbow at a time all the way up to rotate each side of your body. The added rotation will increase the intensity of this movement. Maintain the bent-over position with your chest up and your butt back to ensure that your back remains straight.

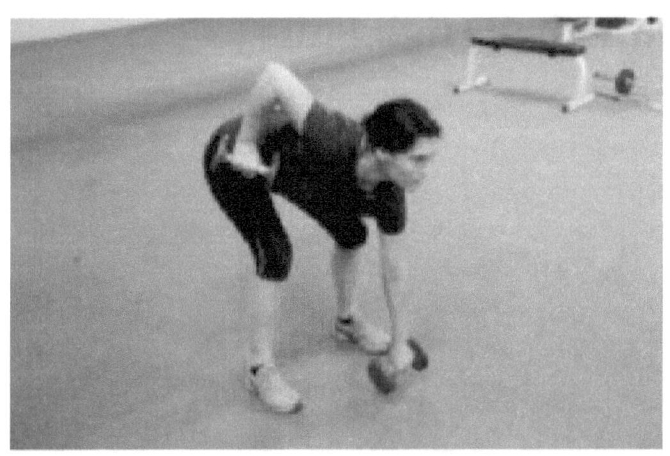

T-Bar Rows

This is another great multi-joint exercise for your lats
and mid-back that also gets the heart rate up. To position
yourself, bend your knees slightly and grab the barbell with
a closed grip. Pull the bar up toward the lower part of your
chest area. Keep your upper body stationary, your chest up,
and your butt out, to ensure that your back stays flat. Note:
Place the end of the barbell in corner, as seen in the picture.

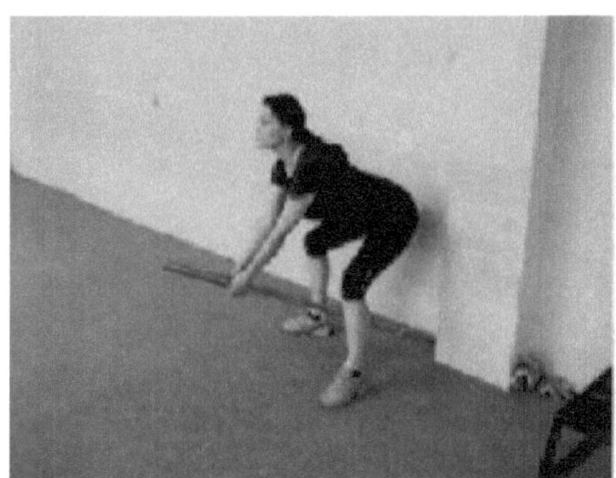

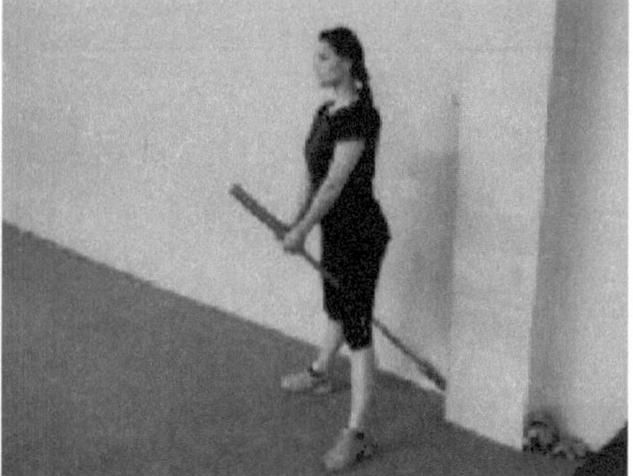

Dumbbell High Pulls

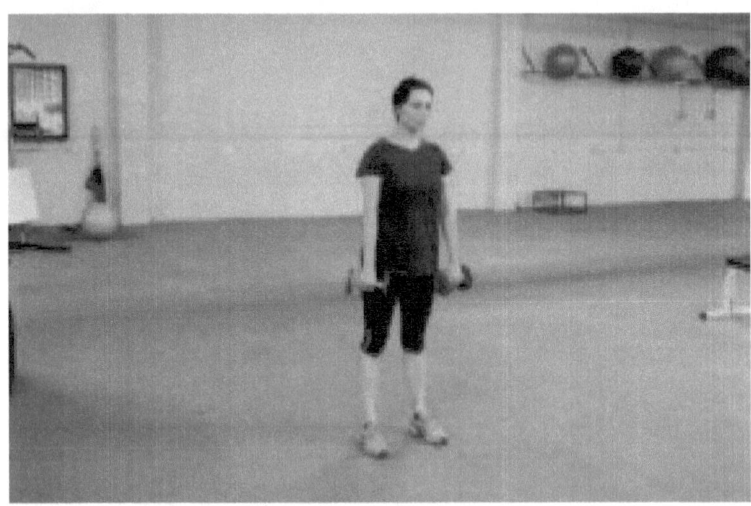

Grab a pair of dumbbells and place them in front of the body. Jump the dumbbells up, bringing the elbows up high and outside. This is a great movement to get you ready for the Dumbbell Cleans. Keep the chest up and look forward at all times.

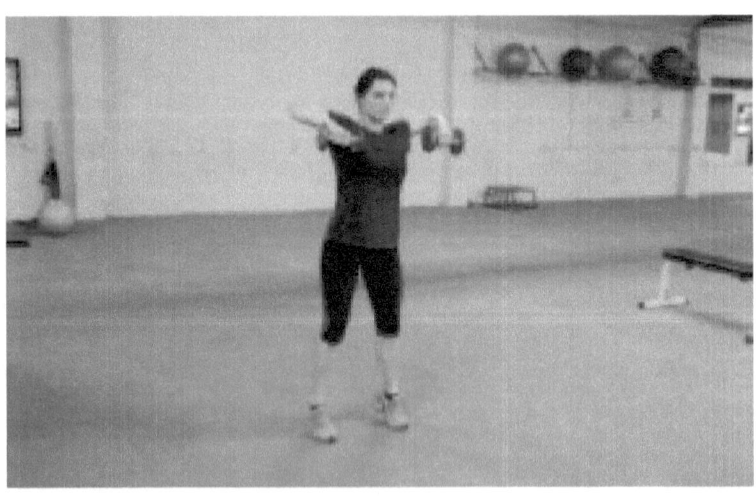

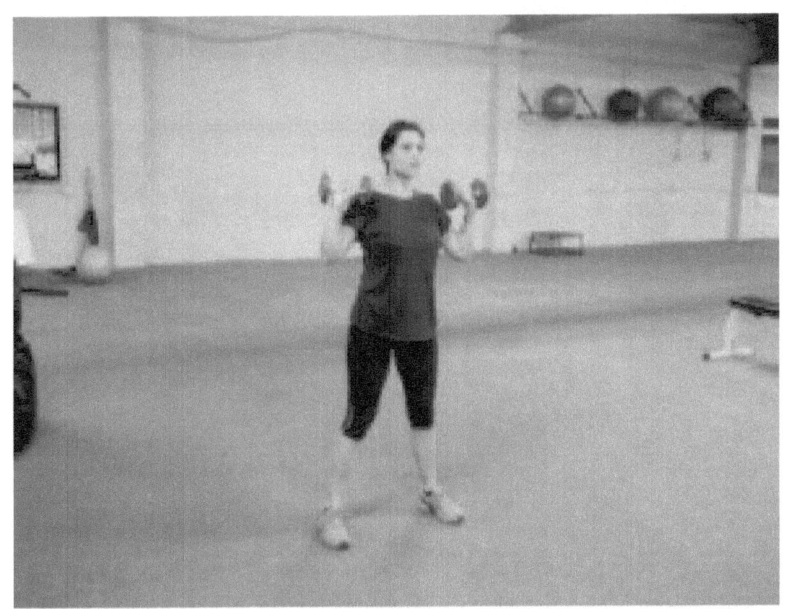

Start with your feet shoulder width apart. To generate energy to get the dumbbells up, dip and then jump the dumbbells up. Use your shoulders in the movement but understand that the energy comes from your legs.

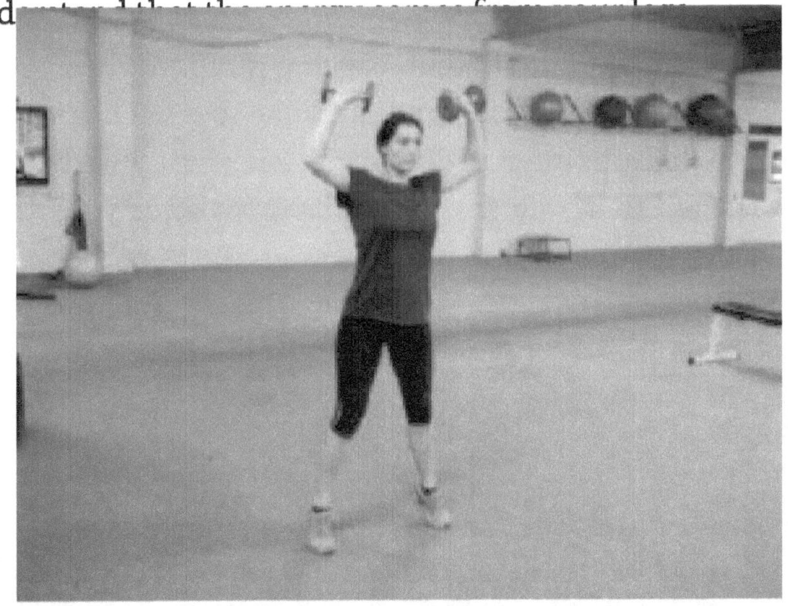

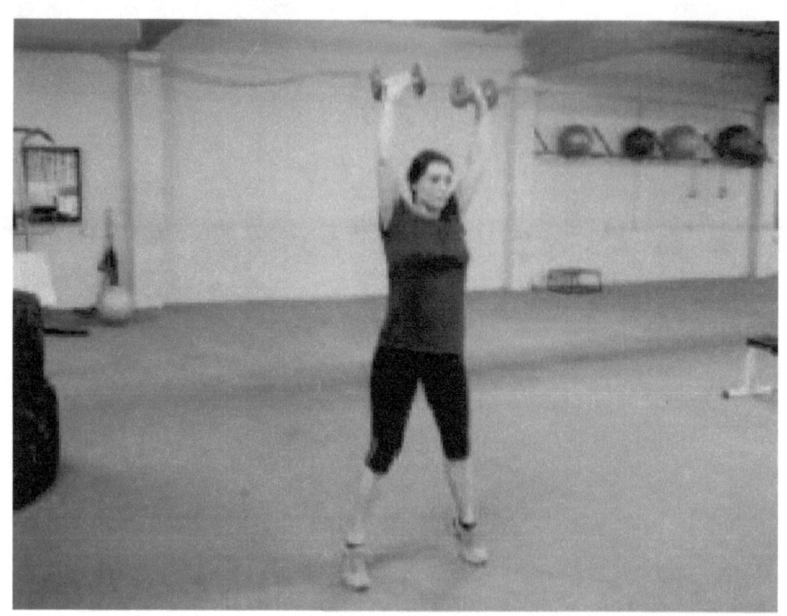

Push Jerk

Similar to the Push Press but finish your movement with a bent leg. Start with a shoulder-width stance with the dumbbells at shoulder height. Dip and jump the dumbbells up by placing one foot out front and one foot back. As you return to the starting position, come back first with the front leg and then follow with the back leg. Keep your arms in line with your ears and push through the dumbbells.

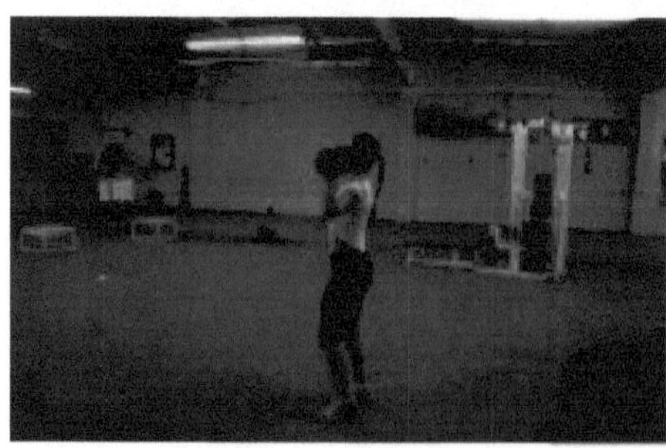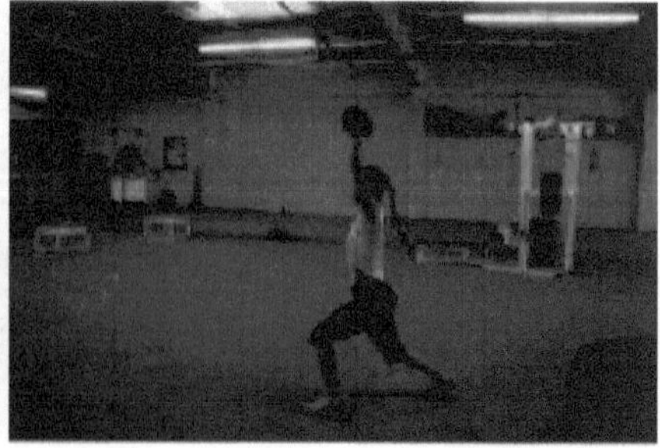

Clean and Jerk

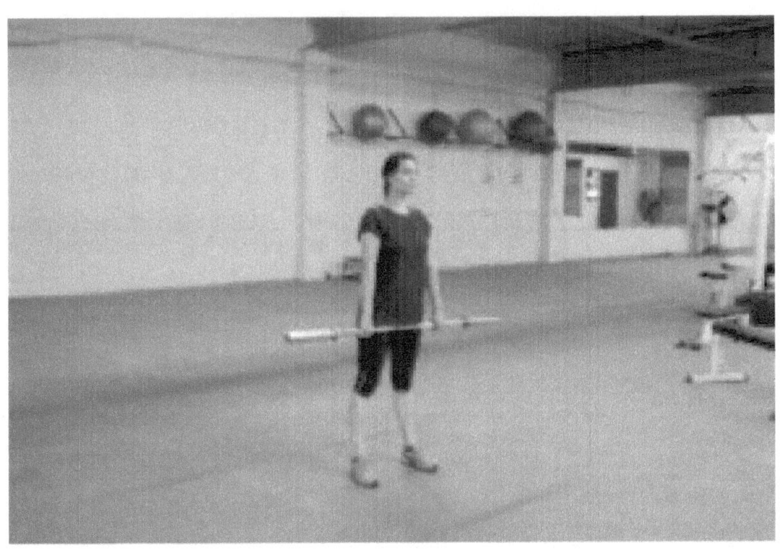

Start with your feet shoulder width apart and the bar hanging at arms' length against your legs. There are two jumps involved in this movement. The first jump brings the barbell to shoulder height and the second jump brings the barbell above your head. On the second jump, split your legs with one in front and the other in back. To bring your legs back to the starting position, first take your forward leg back, followed by your back leg. Continue to repeat the movement.

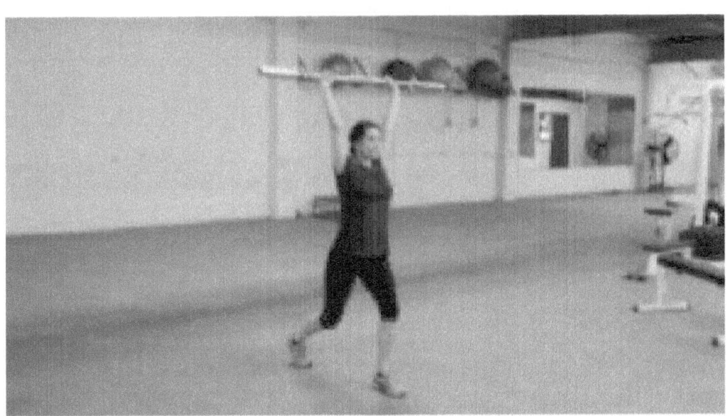

Step-Ups

An exercise that is very transferable to real life. Works one leg at a time and controls the intensity by the height of the bench or by added resistance to your body. To perform the movement, keep the foot up on the bench and press through the heel, ensuring that the glutes come into play. Keep your chest up and look forward while doing your set amount of reps. Switch feet and repeat.

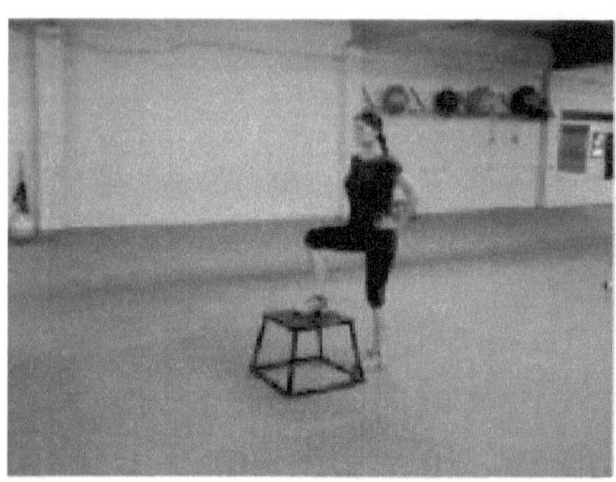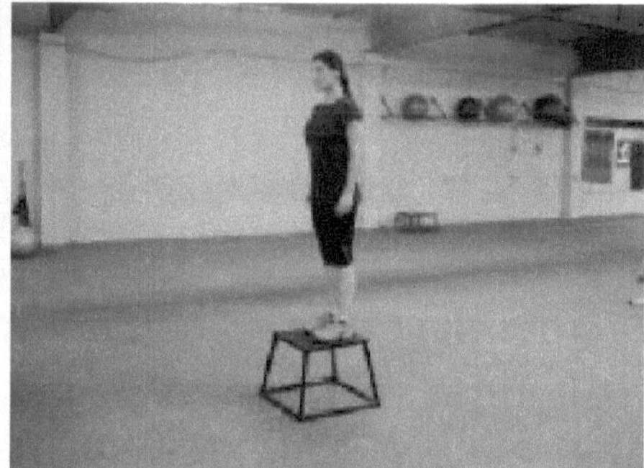

Step-Ups w/ Weight

This is the same exercise as the Step-Ups using your bodyweight, only now you have weights in your hands. Come through the heel of the foot that's on the box. Keep your chest up and look straight ahead. Control your movements coming down and return to the starting position

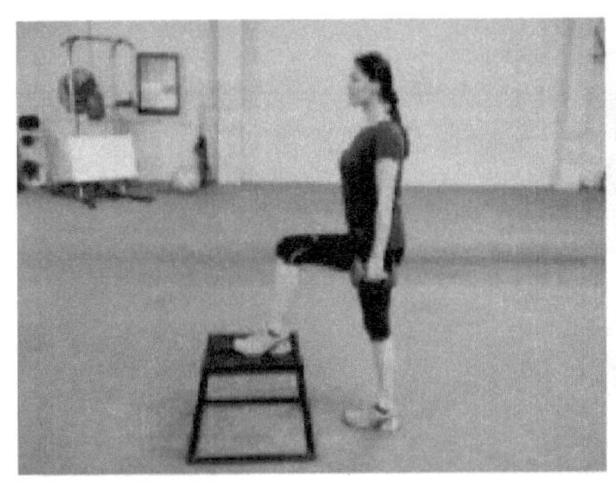 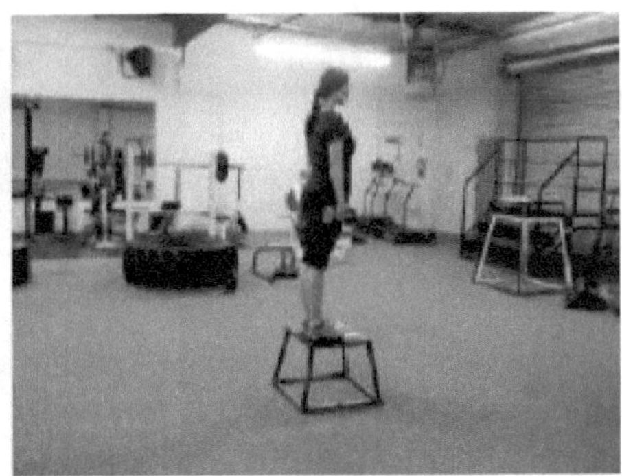

Box Jumps

Start with a shoulder width stance and your chest up. Jump onto the box. Always try to land softly and off your toes. Try to land with your feet flat on the box.

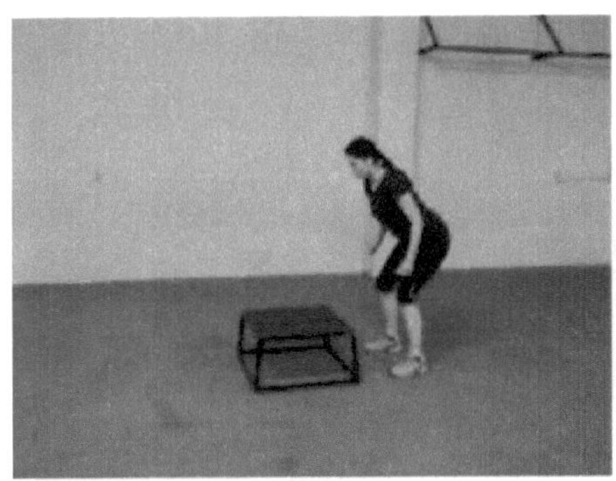 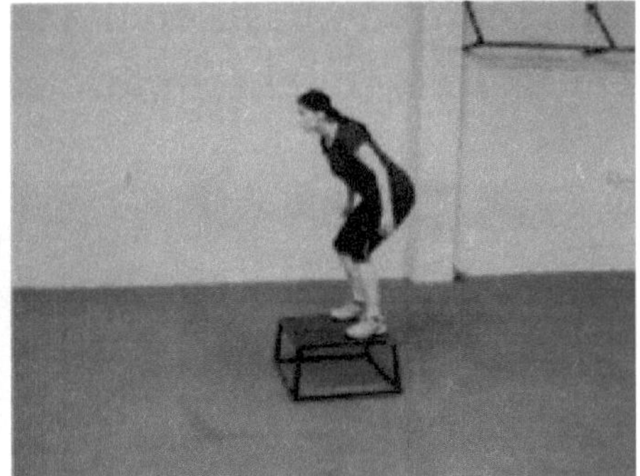

Bear Crawls

This is a great full body, bodyweight movement that works every muscle in the body and burns a lot of calories. It's very hard to beat this exercise for involving so many aspects of the body. Start with your hands and knees and move your body in a controlled manner. We usually start our clients off by moving in increments of 15 to 20 yards.

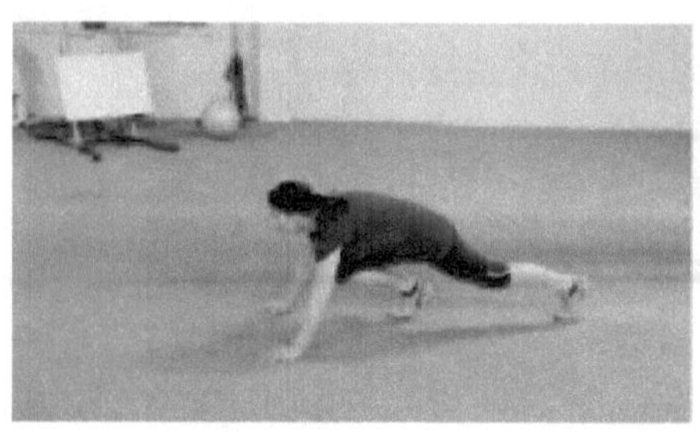 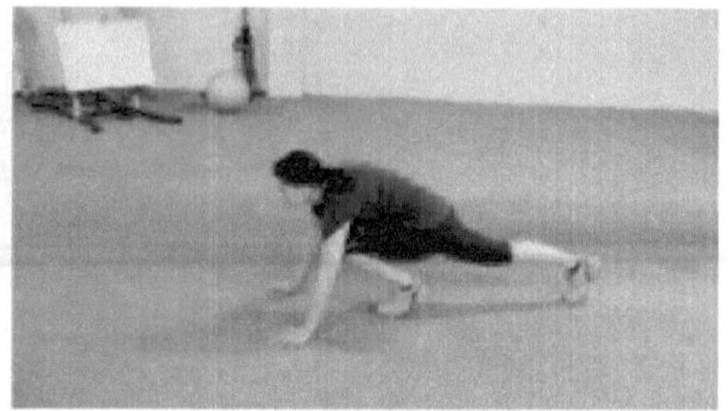

Dips

This bodyweight exercise is an excellent upper body movement that really works the chest, triceps, and muscles of the upper back. Grab the parallel bars or a bench and lower yourself. Press yourself up while keeping your chest up and looking straight ahead. A more upright position puts more emphasis on the triceps, while leaning forward emphasizes the chest muscles.

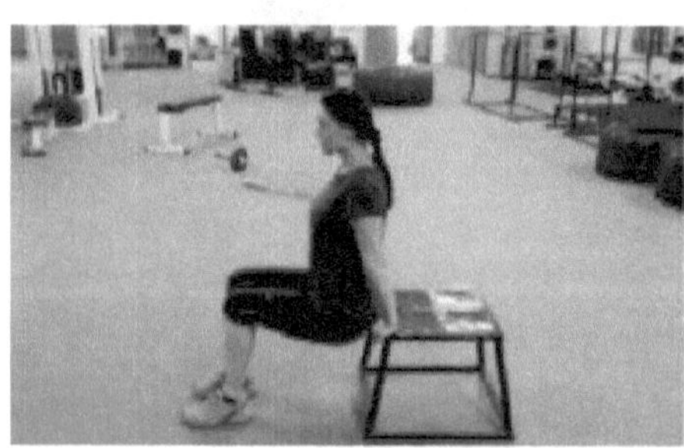 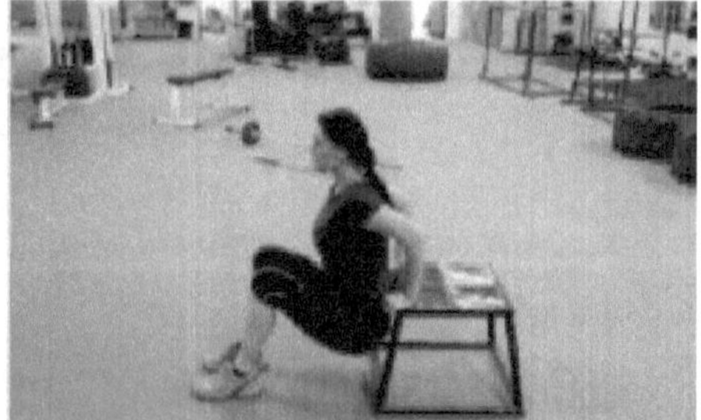

Push - Pull Ups

Place a box right beside the bar and stand on it. Use your legs to push your chin over the bar. Because you're pushing off with your legs, your legs will also be worked in this exercise.

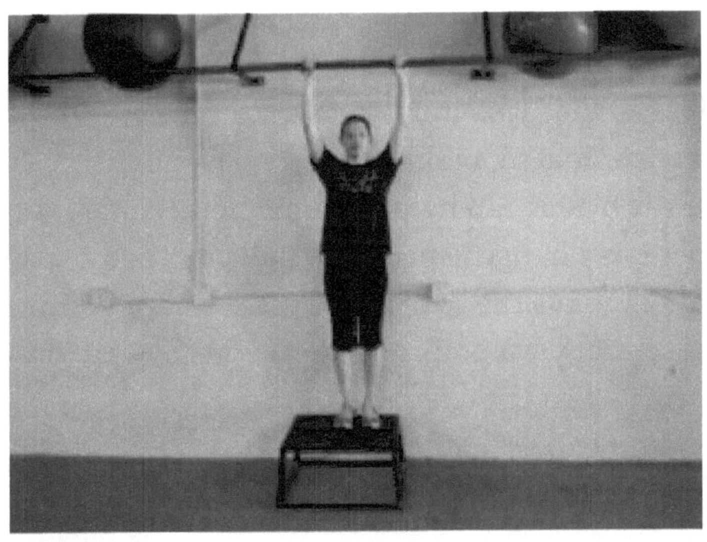

Pull Ups

Incredible upper body exercise. Works the latissimus muscles, shoulders, hand strength, forearms, and biceps. Ability to move is very important with this exercise, and it burns a lot of calories. Start the movement in a hanging position. Pull your body up until your chin is above the bar. Lower yourself in a controlled manner so that your body does not sway forward or backward. Repeat the exercise.

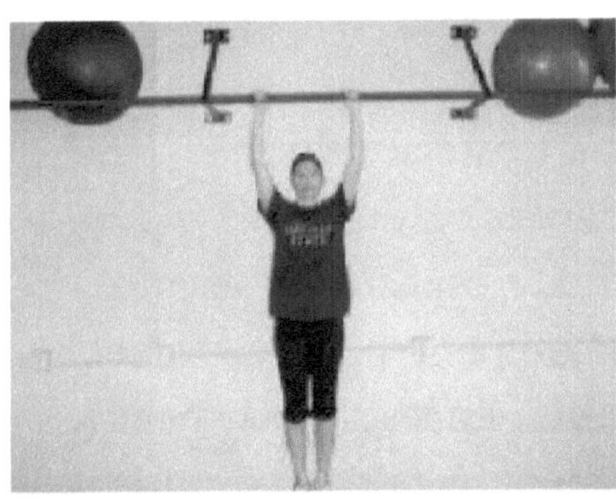

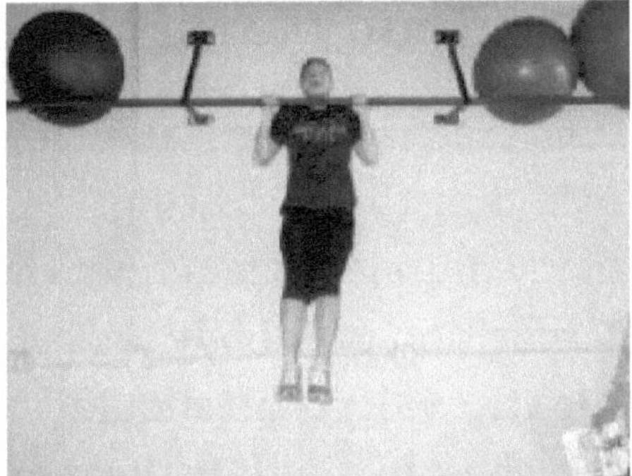

Chin Ups

Chin Ups are the same movements as Pull Ups, except the hands are supinated, making the exercise slightly easier because the biceps can help more efficiently. Start the movement in a hanging position. Pull your body up until your chin is above the bar. Lower yourself in a controlled manner so that your body does not sway forward or backward. Repeat the exercise.

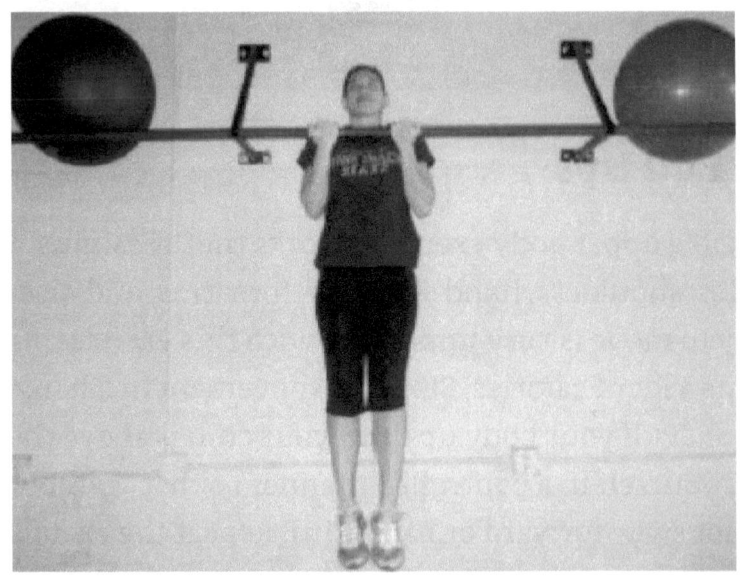

Good Mornings

This exercise is wonderful for the posterior chain, including the hamstring and low back glutes, and works many muscles throughout the body, especially the core. To position your body for the movement, place your feet slightly wider than shoulder width, knees slightly bent, and chest up. Initiate the movement by taking your hips straight back. This movement is very similar to the squat, except you come straight down with the squat. As the hips are going straight back, your upper body will follow. To take your body forward again, squeeze your glutes as you bring your hips forward.

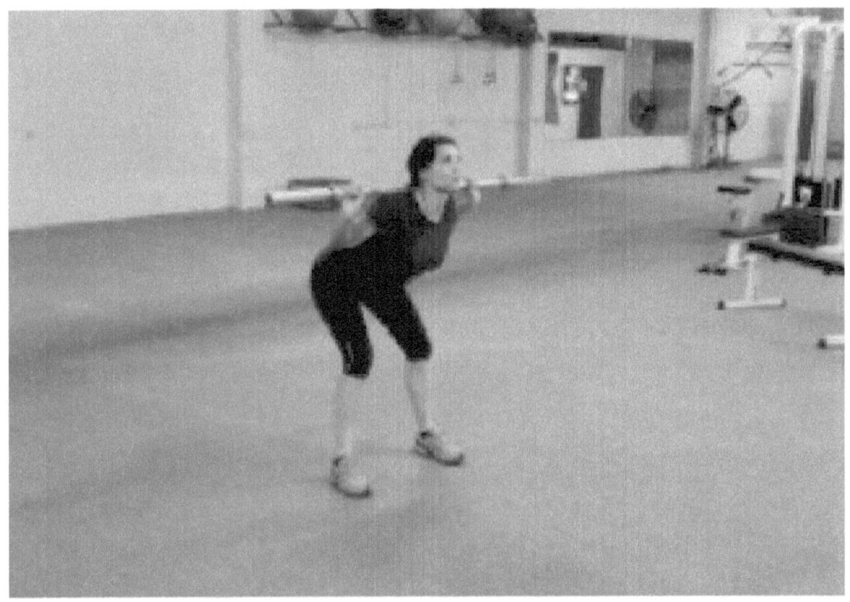

Waiter Walks

This is a great full body exercise, emphasizing the shoulder complex and the core. It also works the ligaments and tendons of the knees and feet, and burns a lot of calories if you walk briskly. Walk with a dumbbell with your arm up in the air and slightly behind the ear. We usually have our clients go for 20 to 30 yards and then switch hands. Always make sure to keep your chest up, look straight forward, and keep good posture.

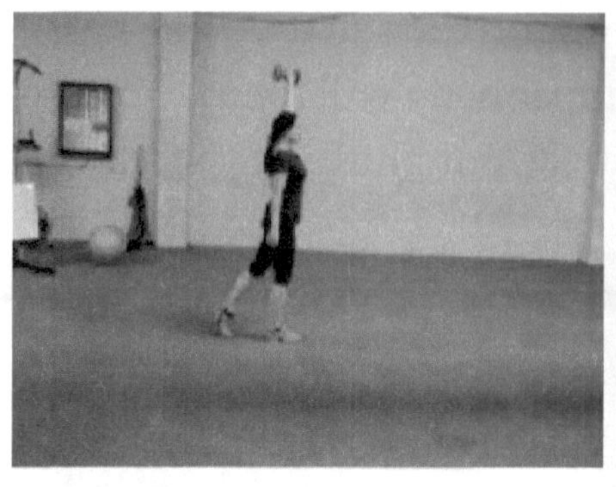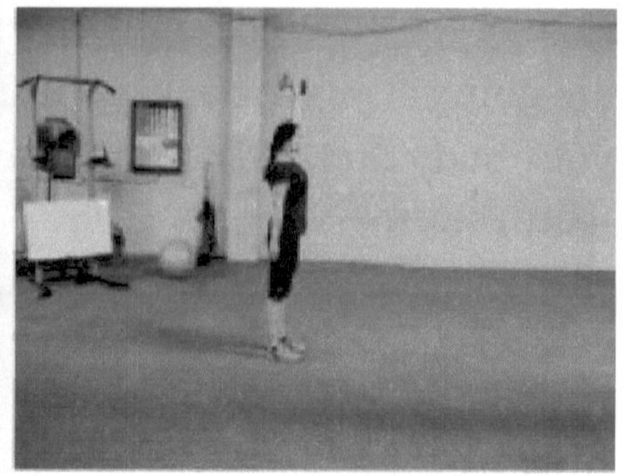

Farmer's Walk

Grab a dumbbell in each hand and walk with your chest up in a good postural position. Look straight ahead and continue walking for 20 to 30 yards. Repeat.

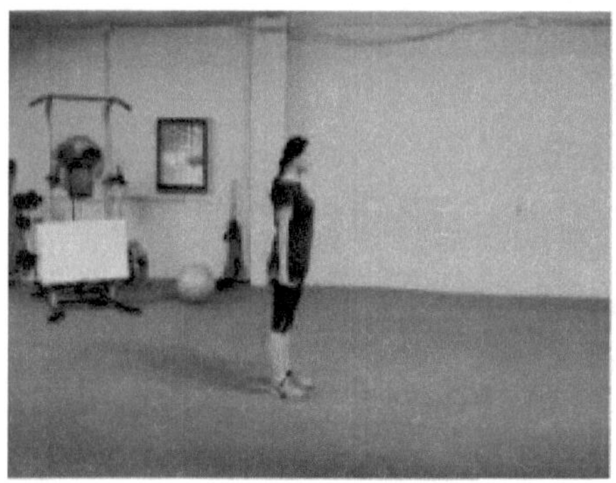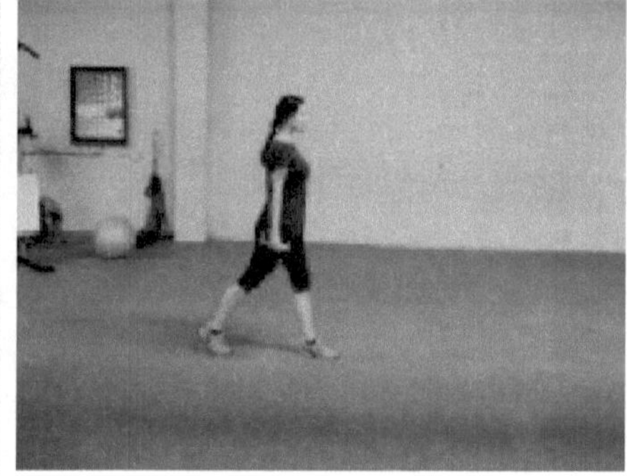

Lunges

Initiate the movement by stepping forward, keeping your chest up, and looking straight ahead. The trailing leg does not have to touch the floor; however, the closer you are to the floor, the more you will activate the glutes. Make sure to keep your upper body stationary to prevent it from drifting forward as you step forward.

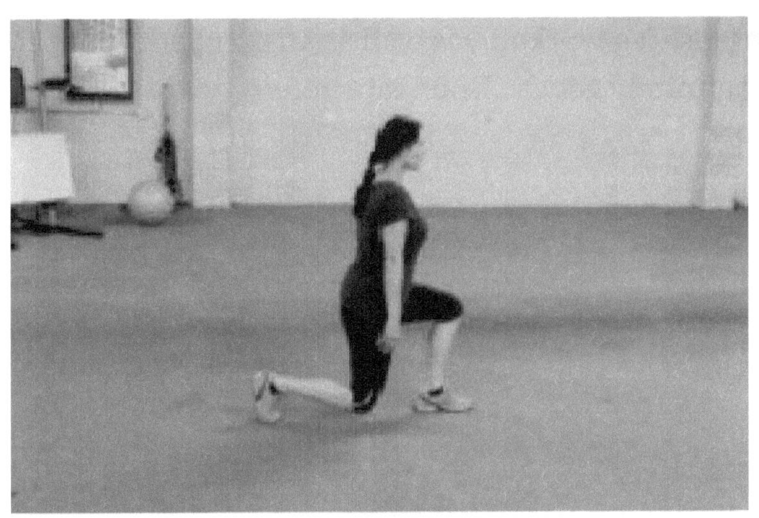

Reverse Lunges

Like the regular lunge, this movement emphasizes the glutes; however, by stepping backwards, it brings a balance challenge to the lift. To perform the movement, stand straight and take a step backwards, bringing the knee straight down. The knee does not have to touch the ground. Make sure that you come through the forward heel when going back to the starting position. Keep your upper body stationary and your chest up.

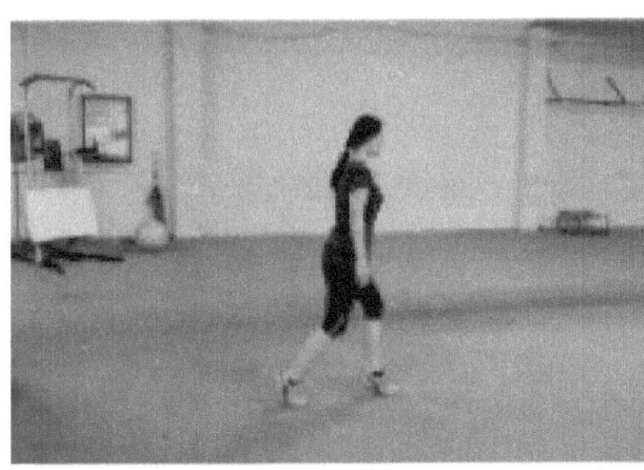 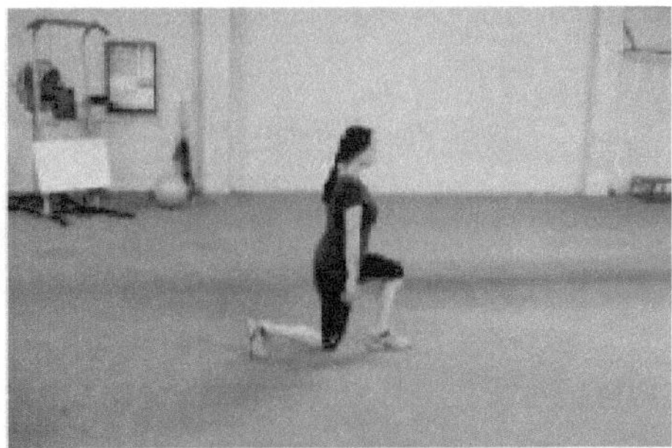

Alternate Split Squats

An intense leg workout, as well as an excellent conditioner. Will definitely get the heart rate up.

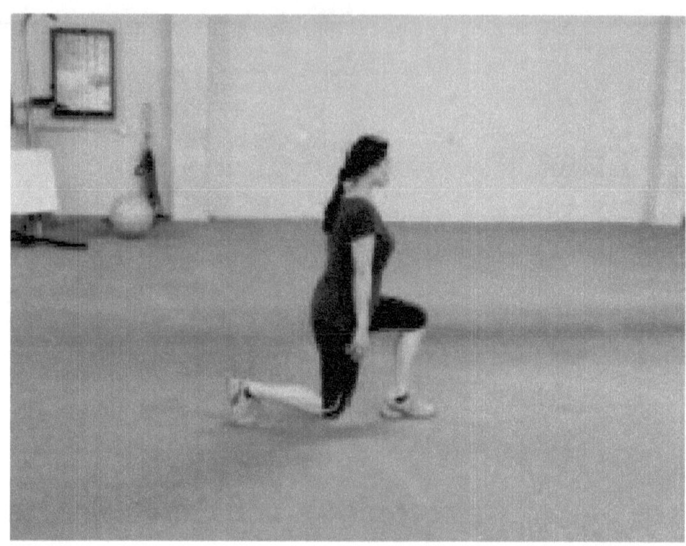

Side Shuffle

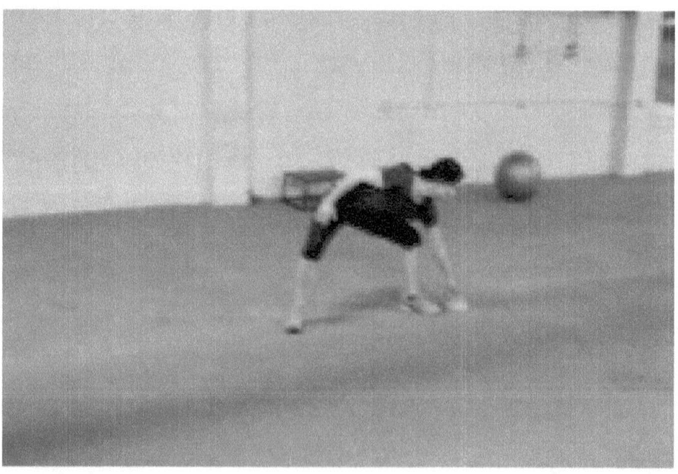

This is a high intensity cardio movement and definitely not a long, slow cardio jog. Perform the exercise by moving side to side and keeping your body low. We usually have our marks set 10 feet apart. Shuffle side to side and repeat.

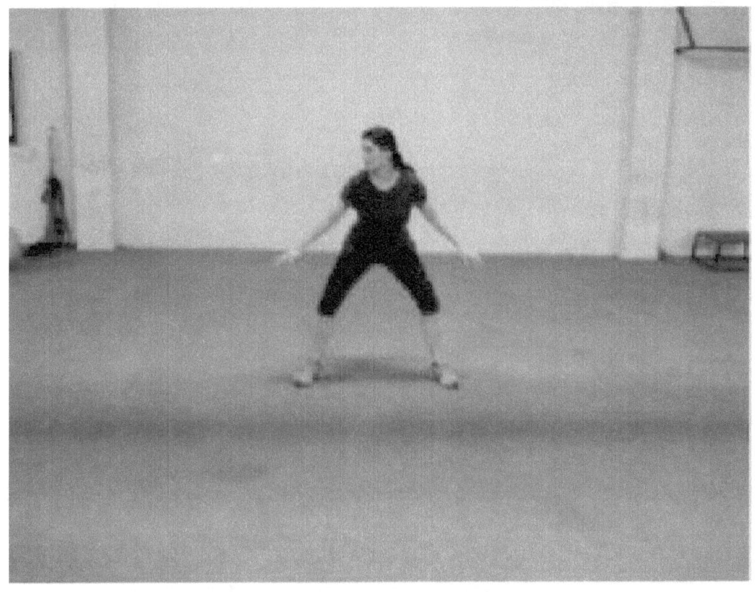

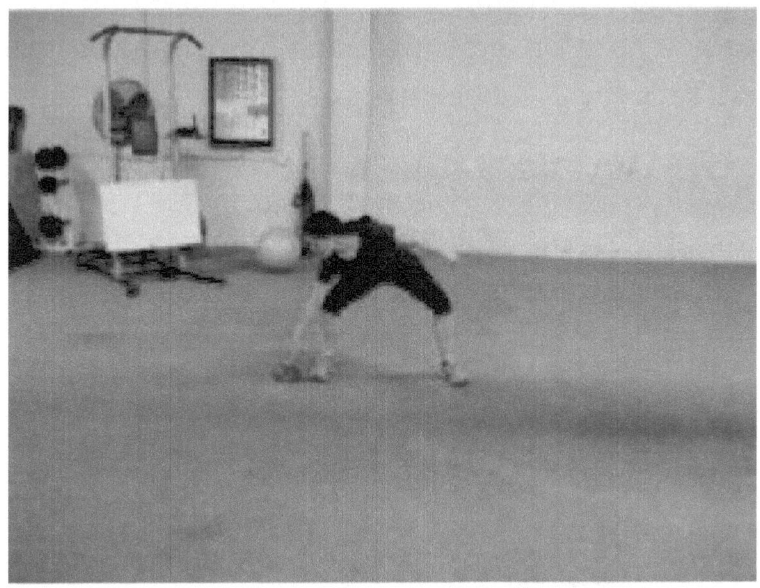

Turkish Get-Up

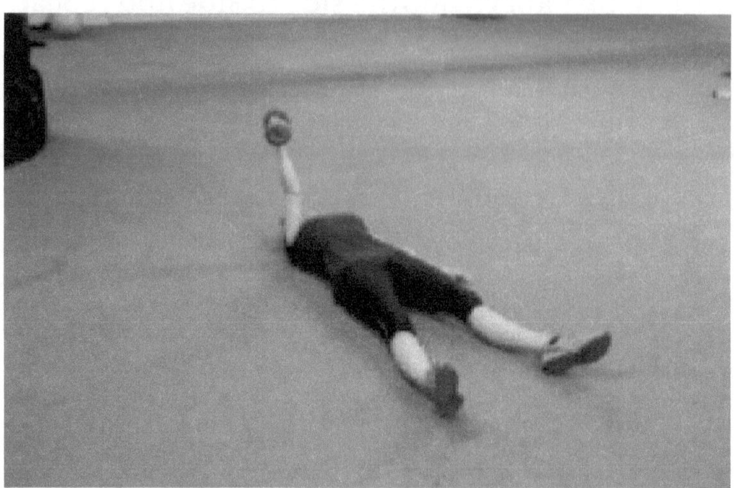

Start by lying down with a dumbbell pressed in the air with one arm. Press through the dumbbell to keep the dumbbell pointed toward the ceiling. As you stand up, either get into a squat position or a lunge position. Throughout the motion, keep the dumbbell pointed up toward the ceiling.

Up-Downs

Start in standing position, then come down into a push-up position. Bring the legs forward and stand up again. Make sure to keep good posture when standing up again.

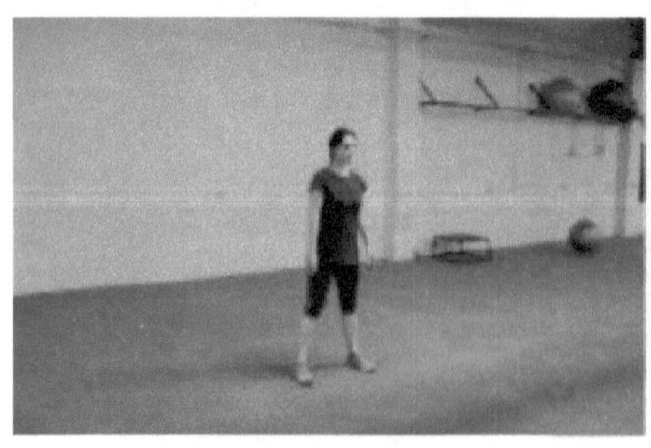

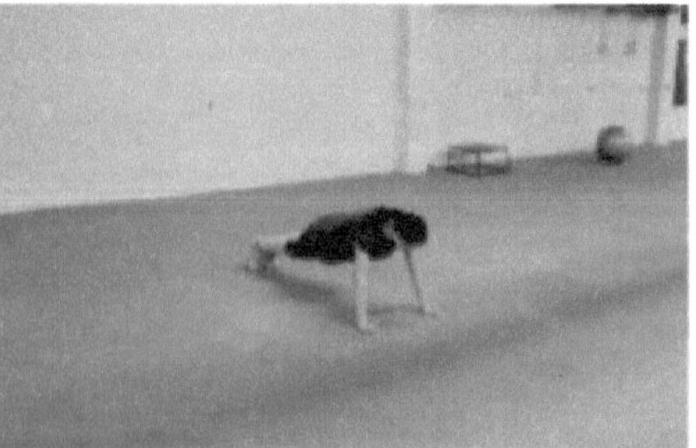

Side Bear Crawls

Start on your hands and feet. With one side of the body, move your arm and leg simultaneously.

Then move the other side. Keep your hips and chin down. Move 20 to 30 yards and then repeat.

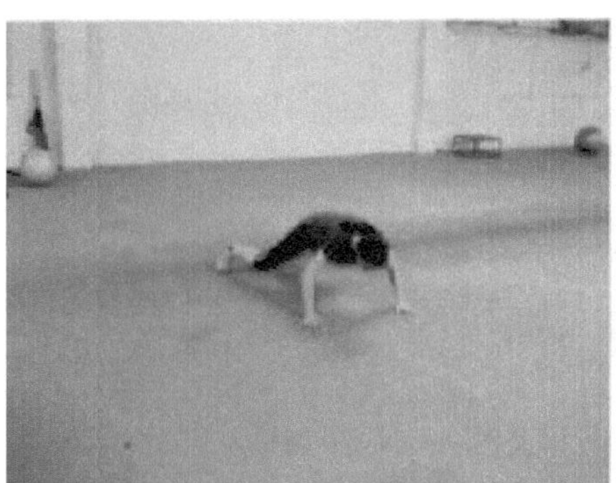 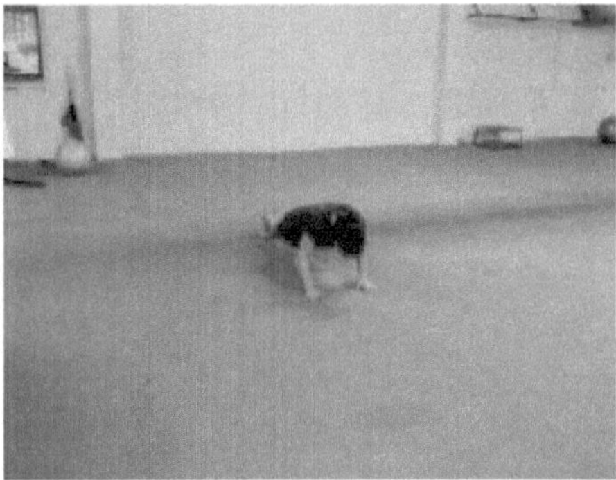

Push-Up

Get in a starting position as the picture to the right illustrates. Keep your hands shoulder width apart. Lower your body down and return to the starting position.

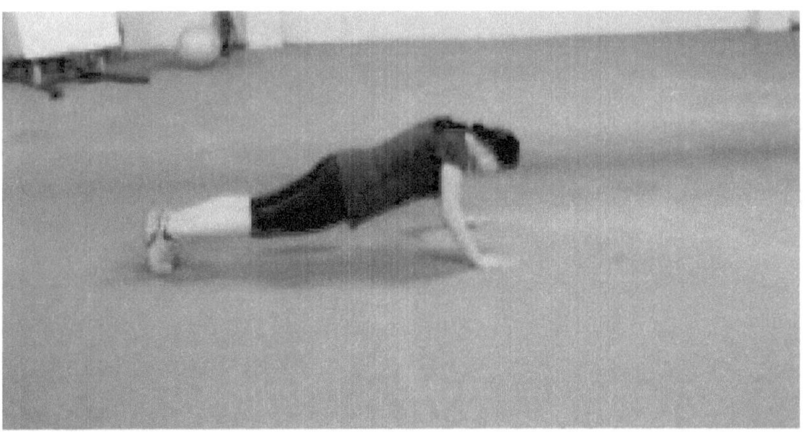

Diamond Push-Ups

To get in the starting position, place your hands close together and let your thumbs and index finger touch to form the shape of a diamond. Lower yourself in a controlled manner and push through the ground, forcing yourself back to the starting position. Repeat.

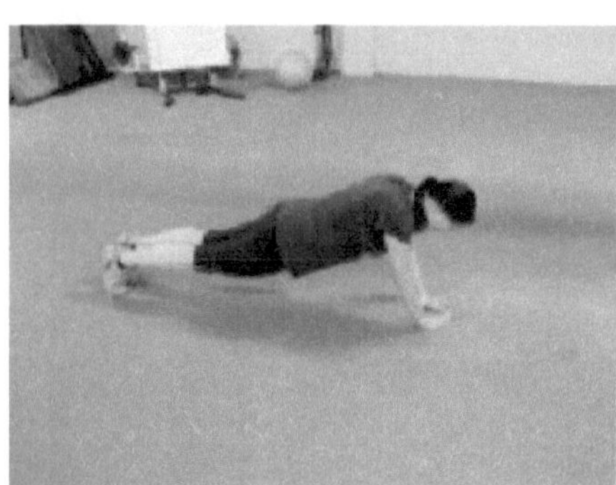
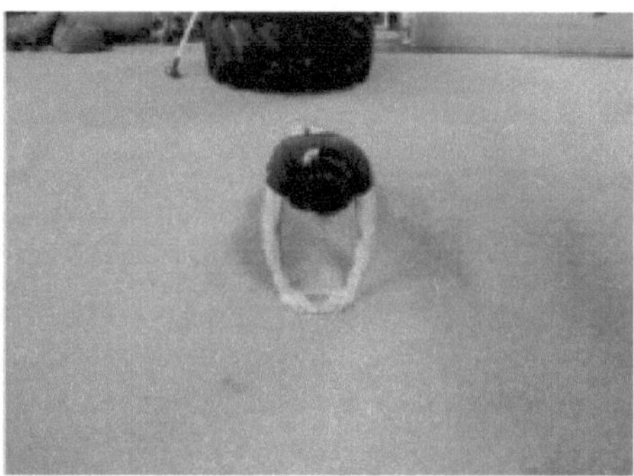

Rotational Push-Up

Get in a regular push-up starting position. Lower yourself down, then when coming up, rotate yourself on one side of the body.

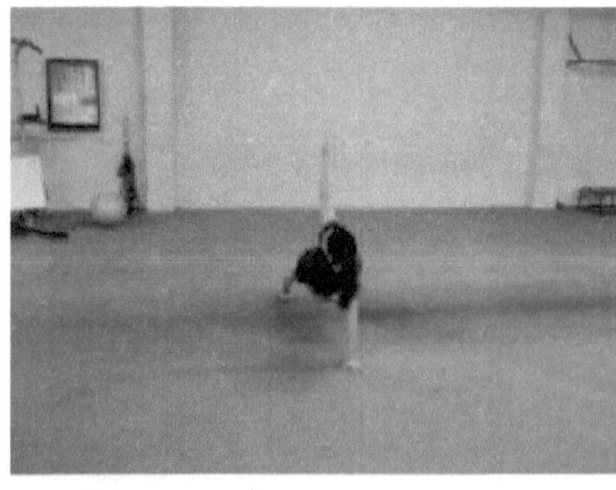
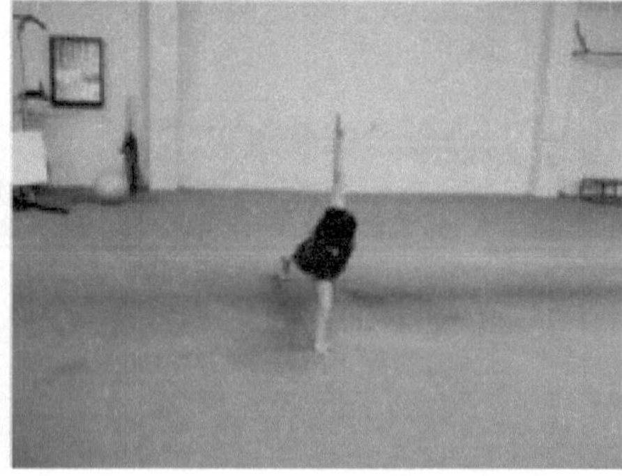

Clap Push-Up

Position yourself as if you are doing a normal push-up. Lower yourself toward the ground and then explode up strongly enough to be able to clap in the air. The clapping motion adds a plyometric effect, thus increasing the intensity of the exercise.

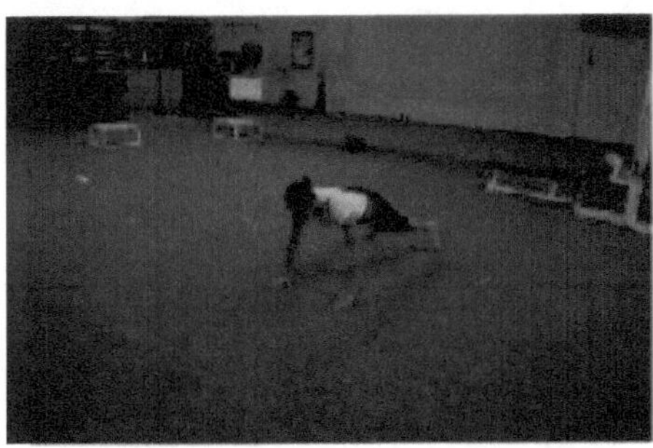 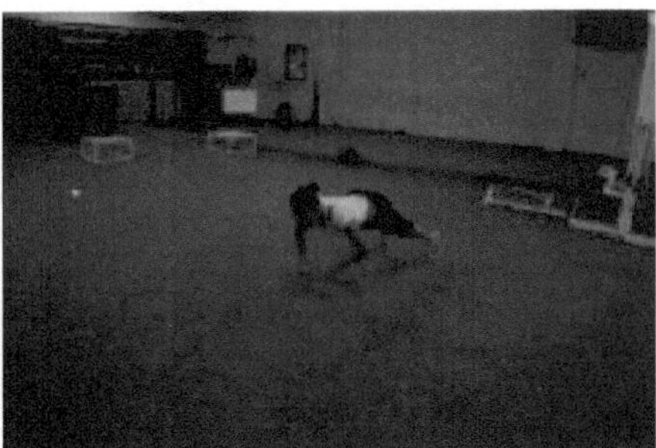

Incline Push-Up

This is the same movement as the regular push-up, only the feet are placed on a higher surface, such as a bench or a box.

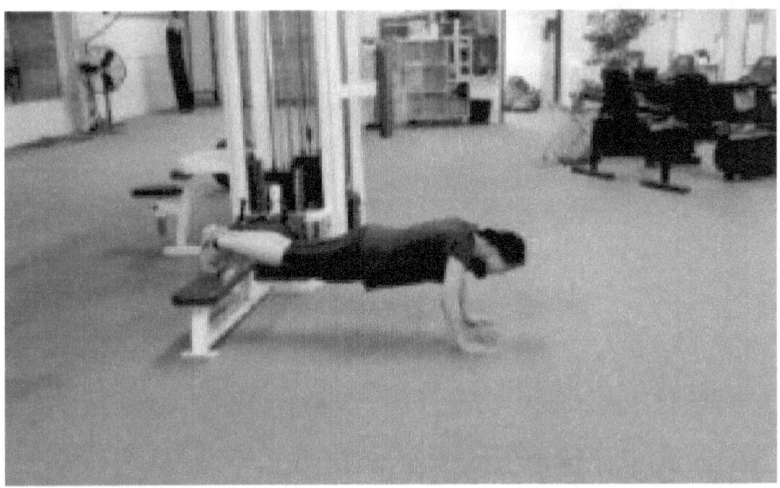

Windmill

Reach into the air with one hand. As the other hand goes down, look up toward the hand that is reaching towards ceiling. Bend your knees slightly. Alternate hands and repeat movement.

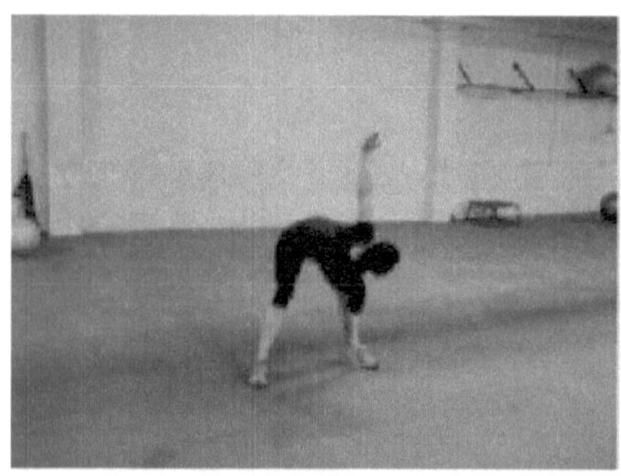 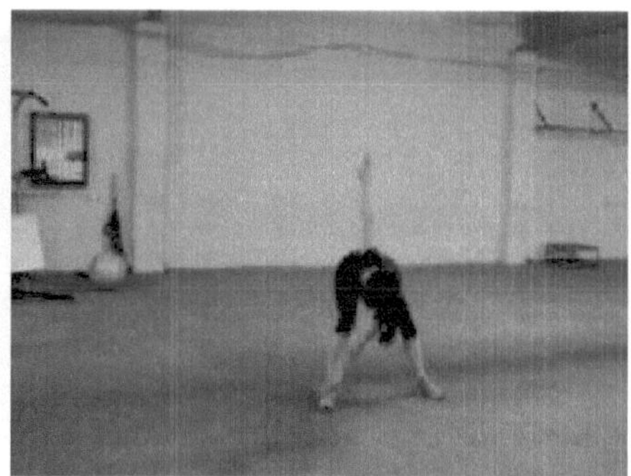

Sprint

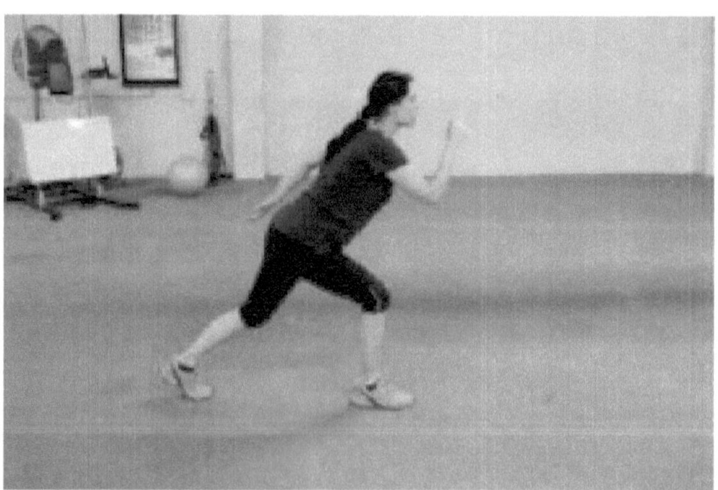

Run 20 to 30 yards at maximum effort.

Dumbbell Russian Twists

Grab a dumbbell with both hands. As you rotate while holding the dumbbell, rotate each foot and keep your arms out in front of your body. Keep your chest up and rotate from side to side.

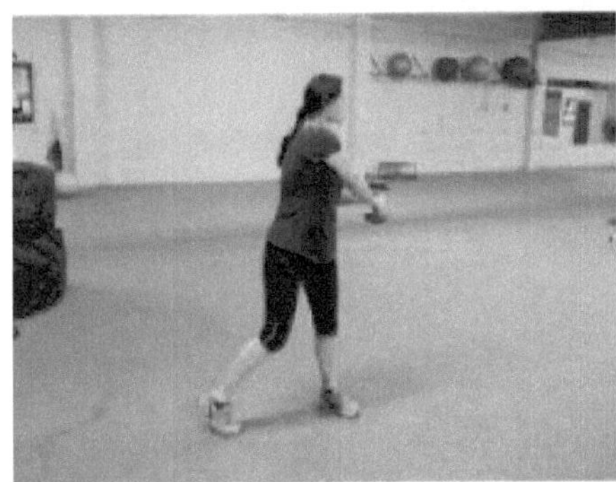 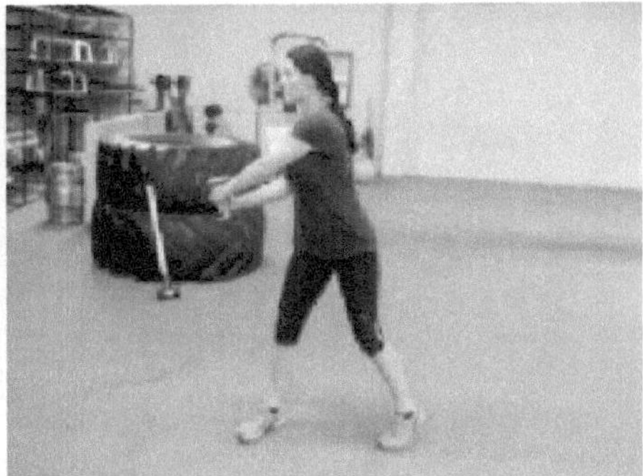

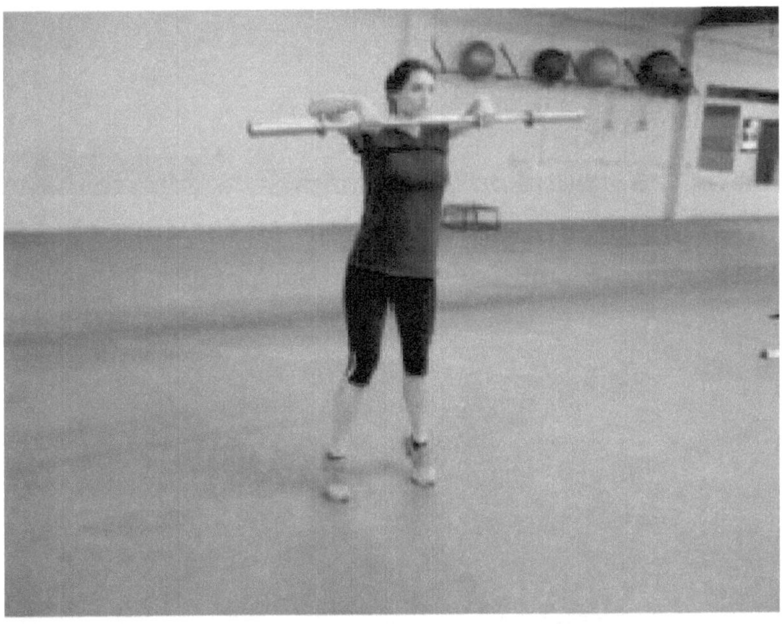

To begin the movement, have the barbell at arm's length

and resting against your legs. Jump the bar up to shoulder height and return to the starting position. Keep your arms straight for as long as you can; keep your arms straight, as when your arms bend, the power ends.

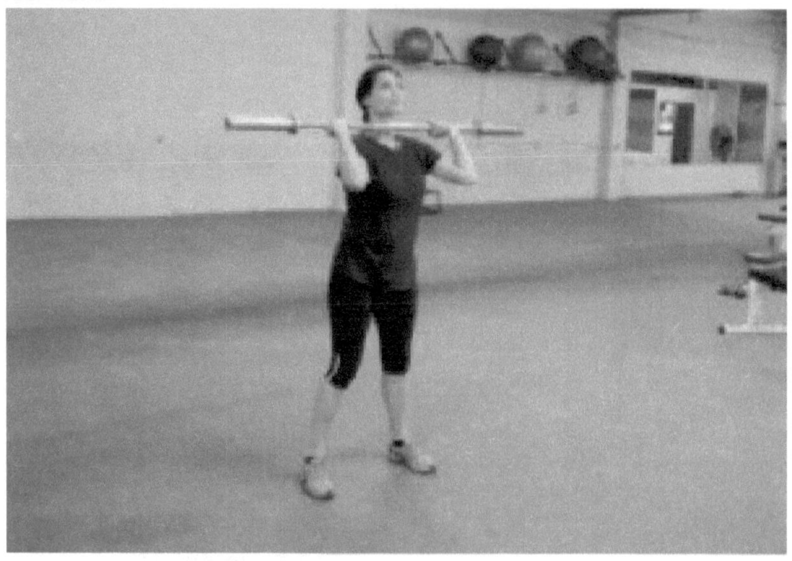

Superman

Lie flat on the ground on your stomach, as you see in the picture. Lift your arms and your legs off the ground and hold the position. Keep your chin down at all times.

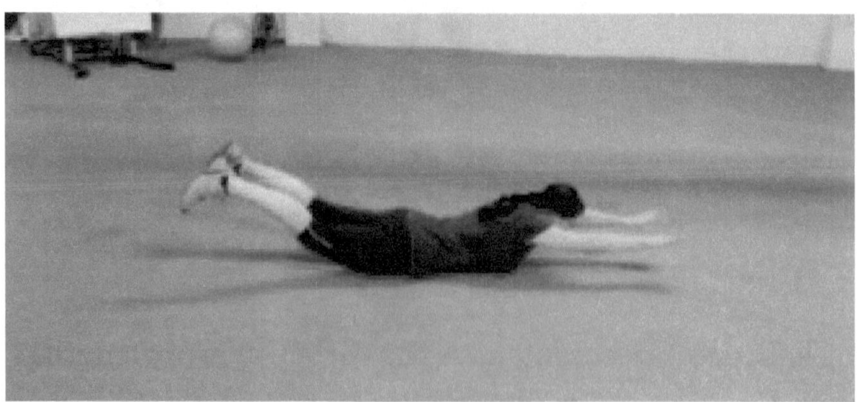

Beginner's Recline Pull

To position yourself, place yourself under the bar as shown in the pictures, with your feet on the ground. To perform the movement, squeeze your glutes to keep your hips up. Pull your chest straight up to the bar while focusing on coming straight up to the ceiling.

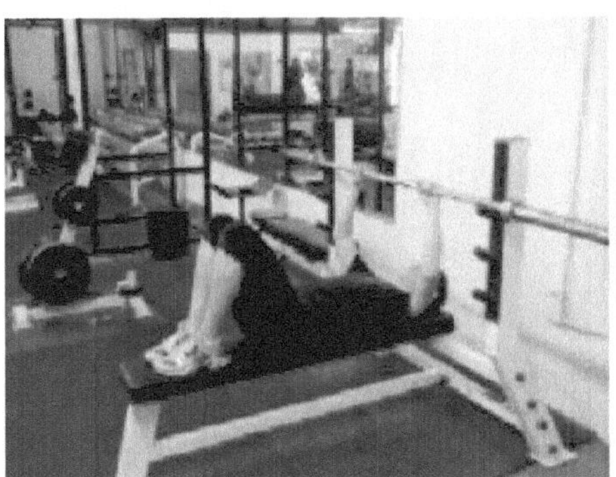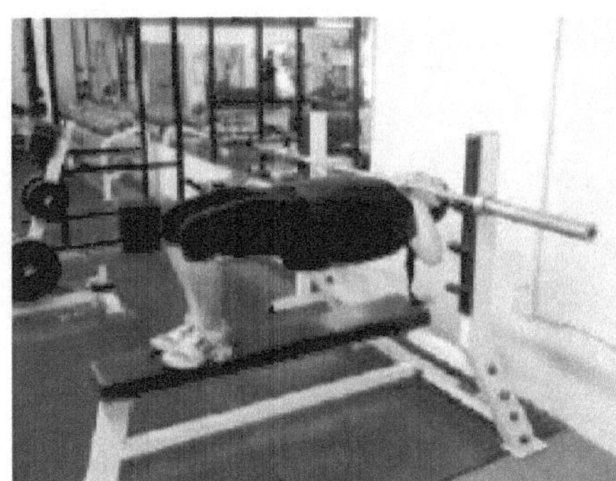

Recline Pull Ups

The recline pull up is a great exercise to work up to regular pull up. Also works upper back and shoulder muscles very well.

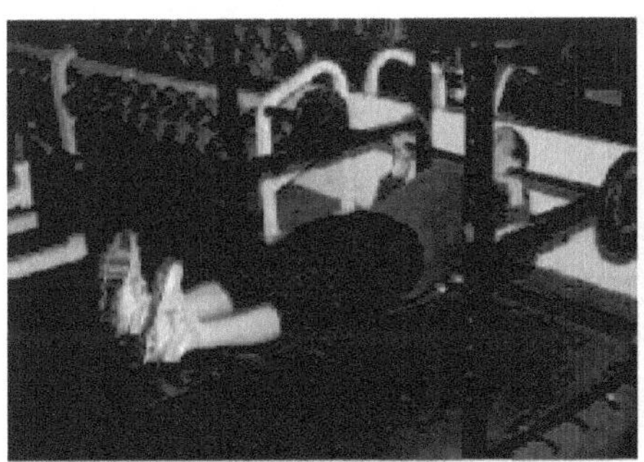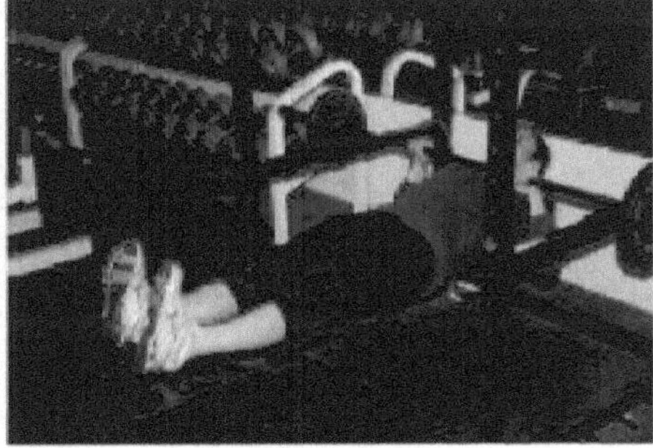

Barbell Shovel

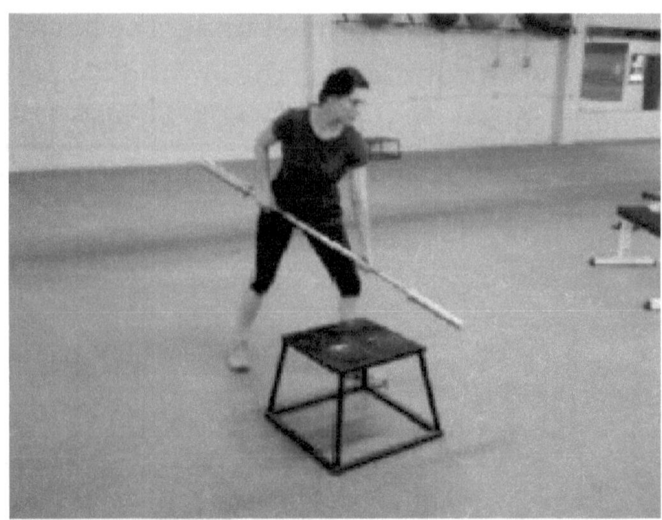

Grab a barbell. The closer you put your top hand to the end, the more control of the barbell you will have. The farther away the hand is, the more difficult this movement becomes. Move the barbell from one side of the box to the other, making sure that you bend your knees with each step. Make sure that you lift the barbell over the box when going from side to side.

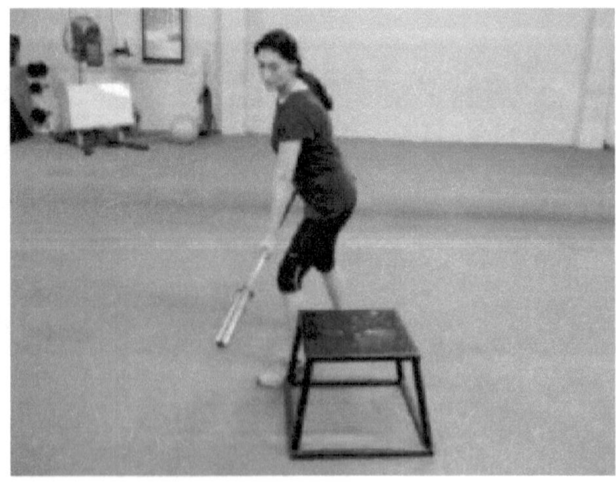

Crab Walks

To perform this movement, get on your hands and feet, as seen in the pictures. Move forward about 15 to 20 yard then move backward to the starting position.

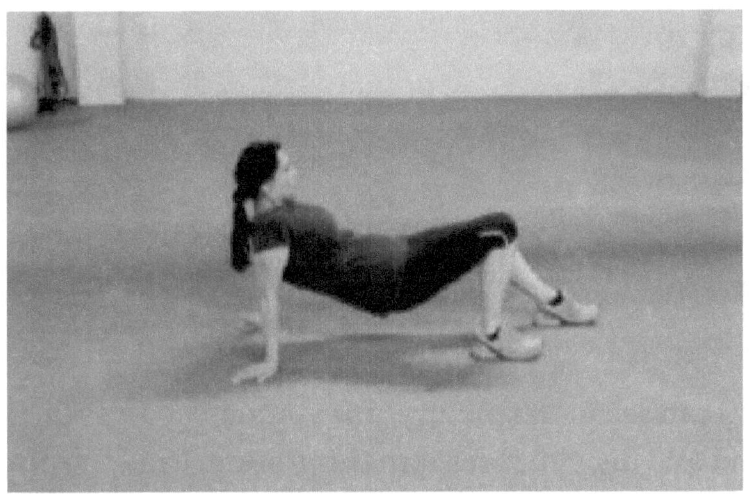

Bus Drivers

To perform the exercise, grab a barbell and place one end of it on the floor, as show in the pictures. Rotate the barbell from side to side, keeping the arms straight ahead while looking straight. Each time the bar goes from one side to the other side, rotate with the trailing leg.

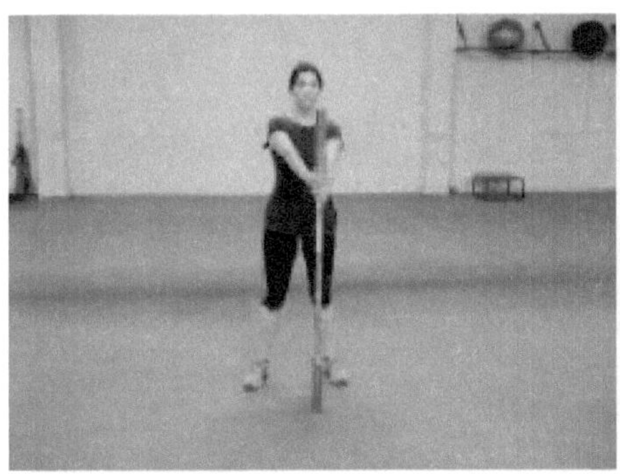 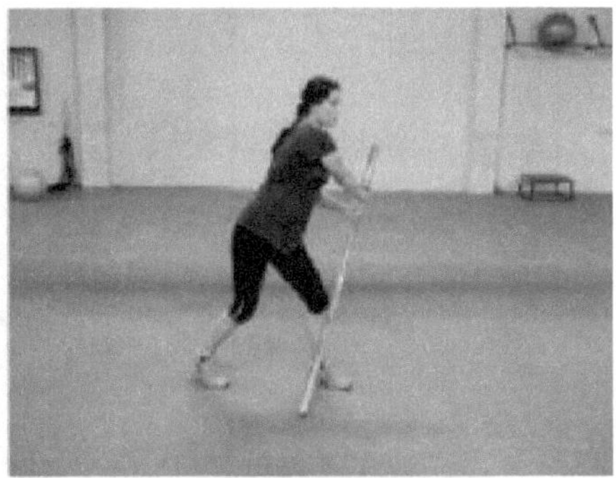

Plank

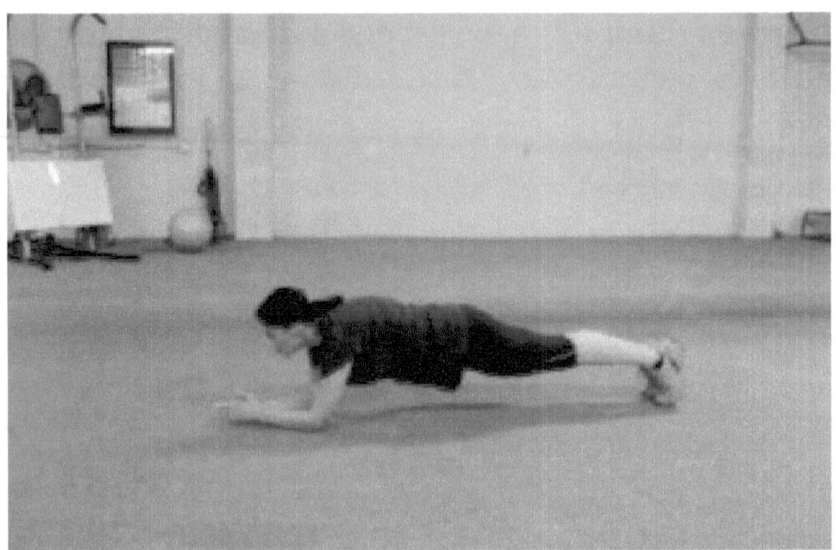

As you can see in the picture, put your lower arms on the ground and dig your toes into the ground. Hold the position for as long as you can.

Side Planks

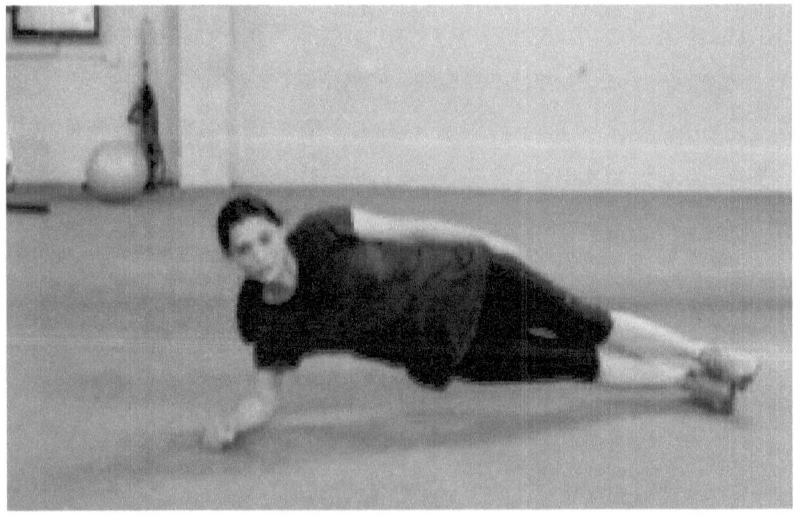

This movement is similar to the plank except that your body lies on its side with your arm supporting it. Hold the position then switch to the other side.

Rotational Planks

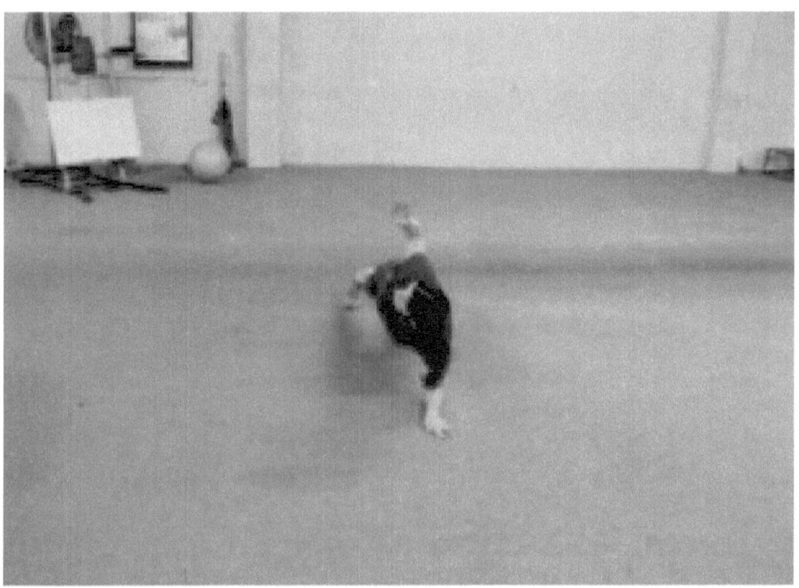

Start position as a regular plank and rotate from side to side until one arm is lined up with the other arm.

Criss Cross Jumping Jacks

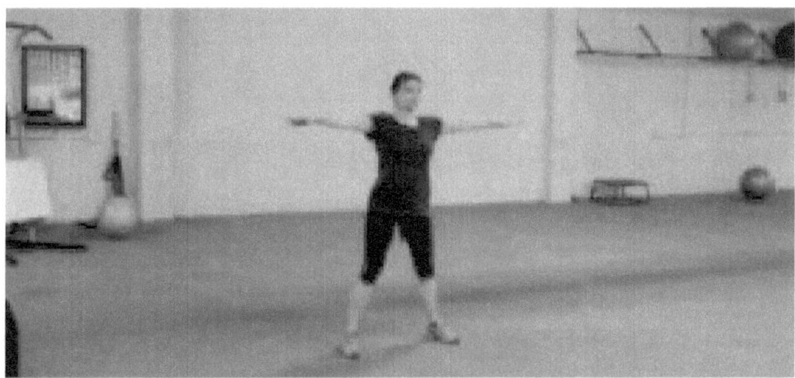

This movement is very similar to regular jumping jacks except that your arms are in front of you, moving over and under each other. Your legs are also criss-crossing each other in the front and in the back of your body.

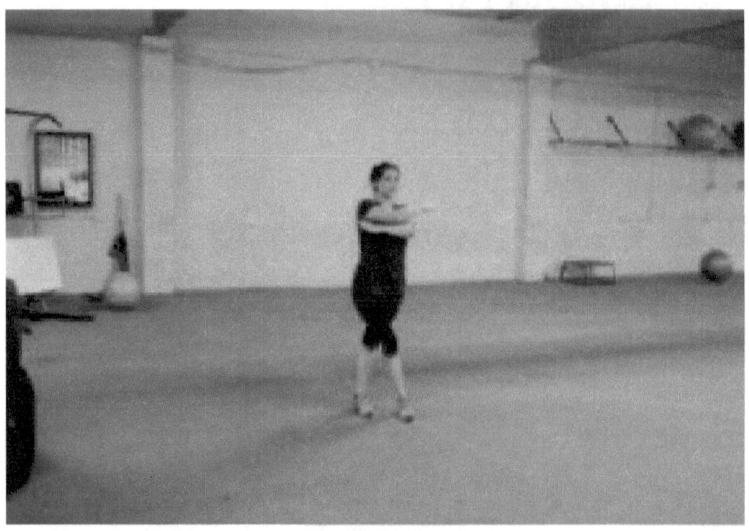

Mountain Climber

Start in an upright position. Stagger your legs, with one foot in front of the other. Have your hands on the floor, shoulder width apart. Start the movement by shifting your legs forward and backward in a rapid motion.

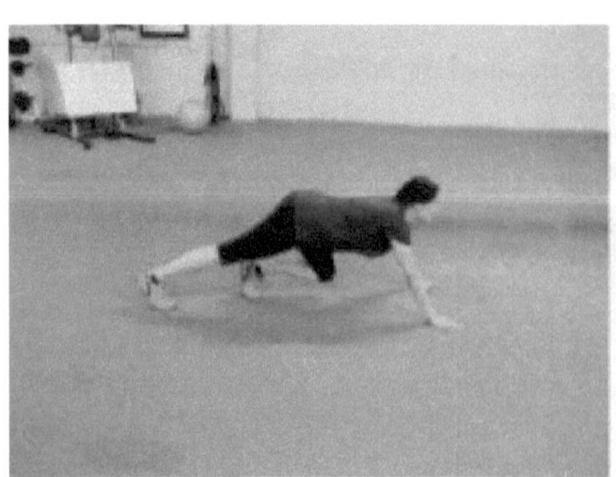 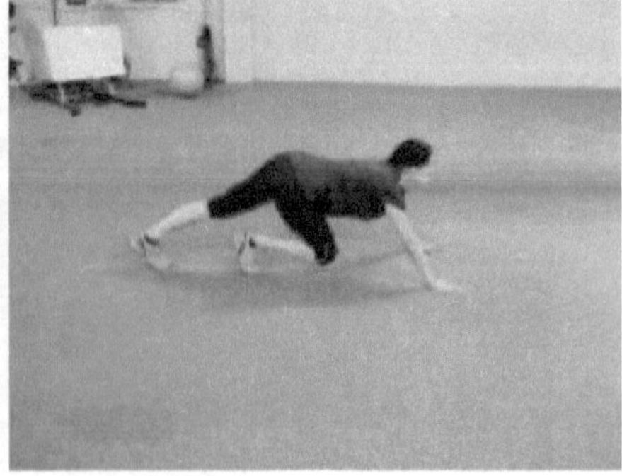

Dumbbell Swings

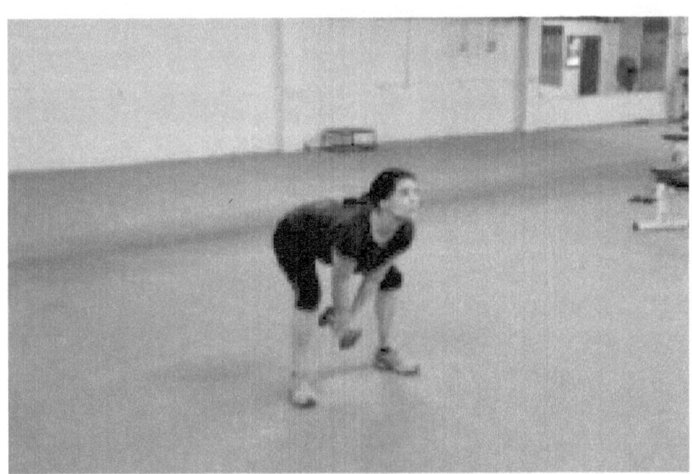

The dumbbell swing is done by swinging the dumbbell between your legs and bringing it to eye level to start. Later on, we'll bring the dumbbell overhead. This exercise really works the hamstrings, glutes, and lower back. These exercises are also known for working the posterior chain.

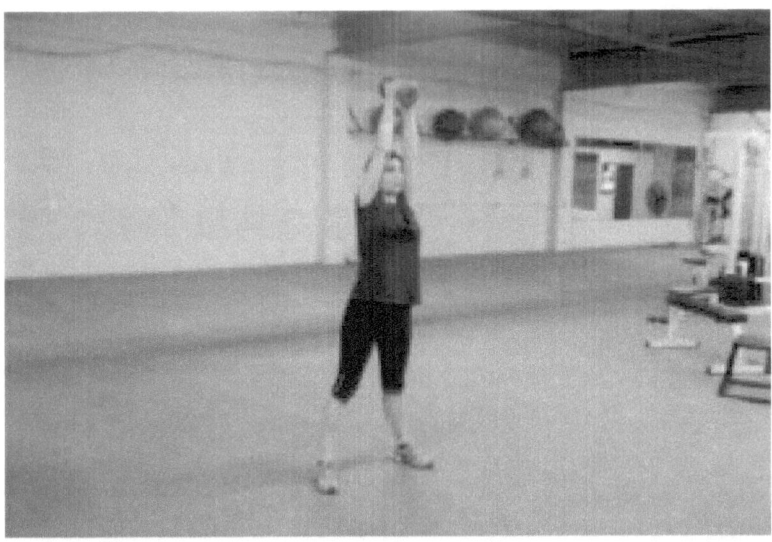

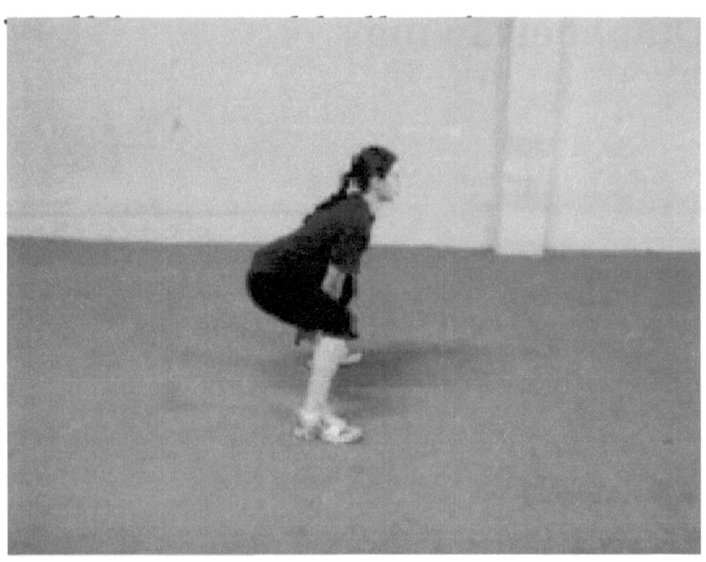

This is the same movement as the regular dumbbell swing, only now we add a step. When the dumbbell is weightless in the air, take a step forward. Alternate each foot forward, and walk with the dumbbell for 10 to 15 yards then return to the starting position.

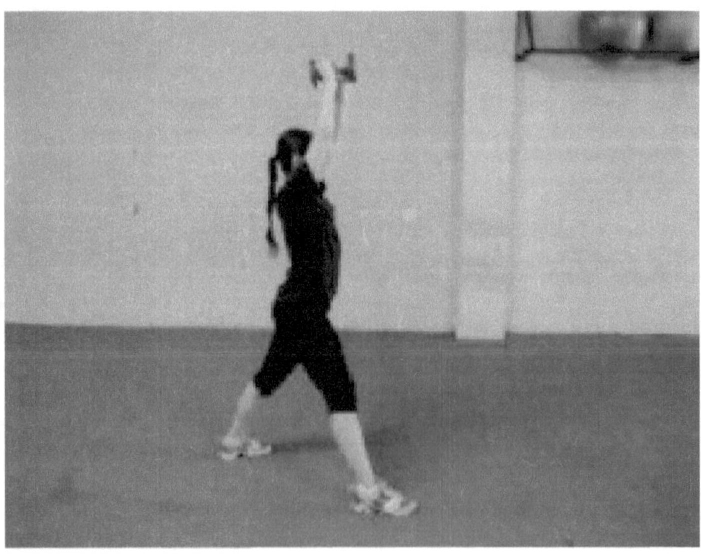

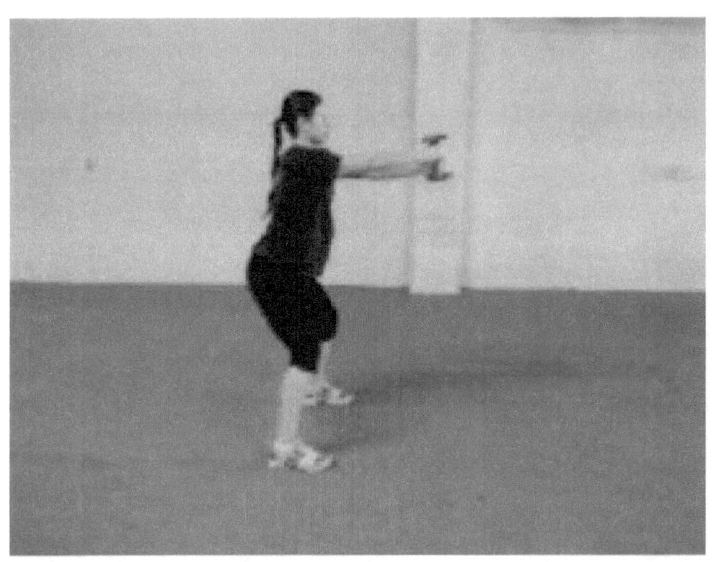

Lateral Dumbbell Swing

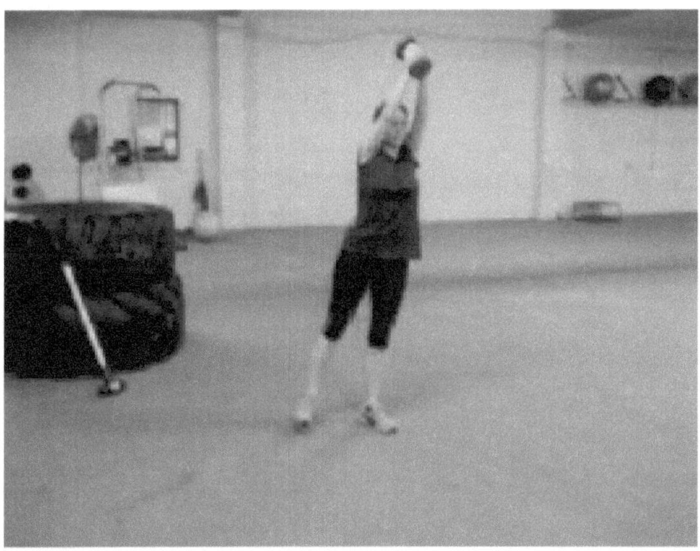

This is the same movement as the regular dumbbell swing, only now we add a lateral side step. As the dumbbell is rising, take a step toward the other foot then return to the starting position.

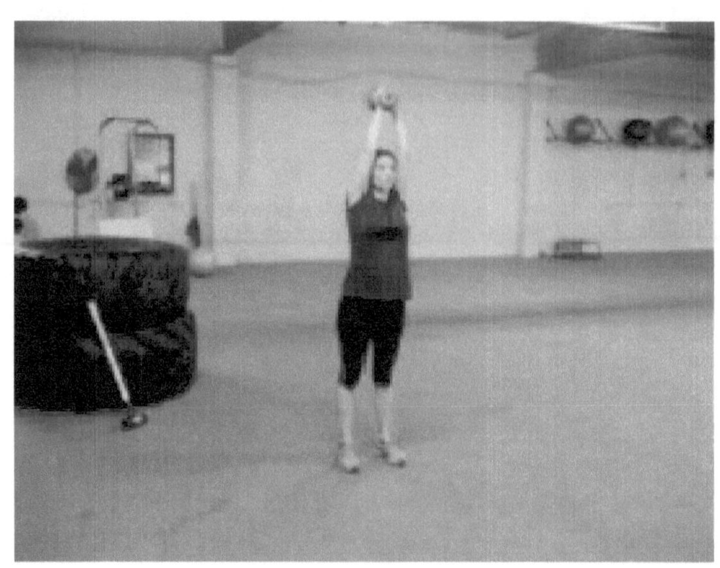

Barbell Snatch

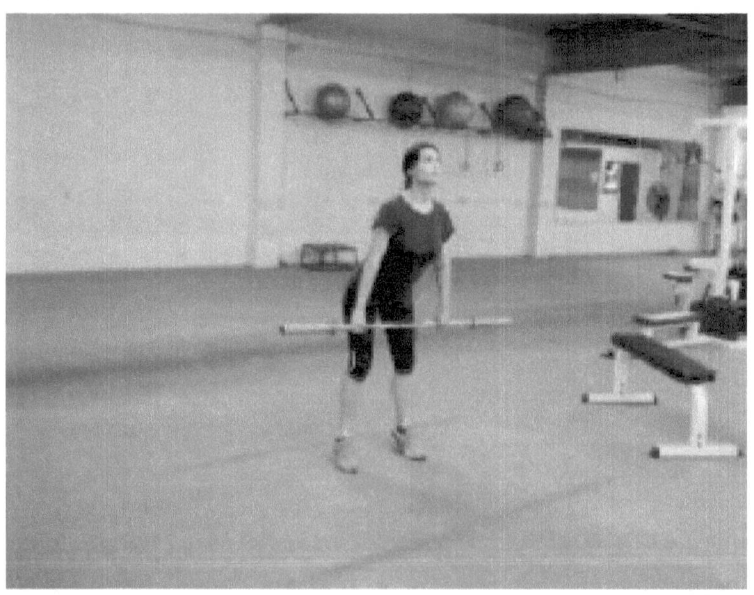

Start with your feet shoulder width apart and the barbell hanging at arm's length. This movement requires one jump to get the barbell above your head. When the barbell is above your head, make sure you push through the barbell to keep it in place. Return to the starting position and repeat.

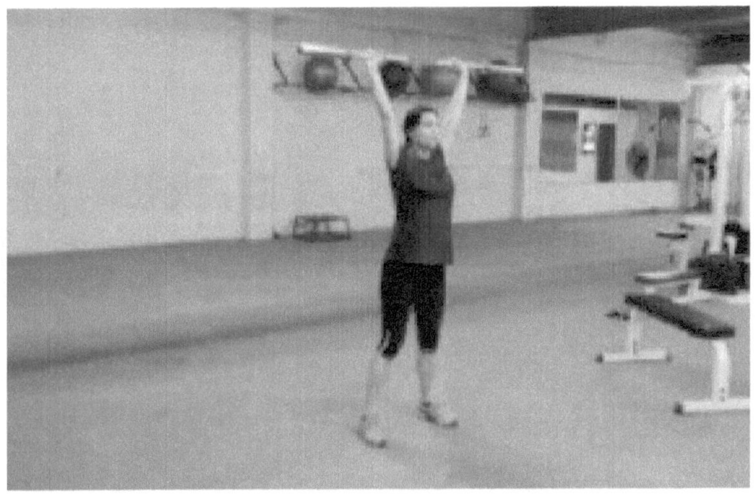

Dumbbell Snatch

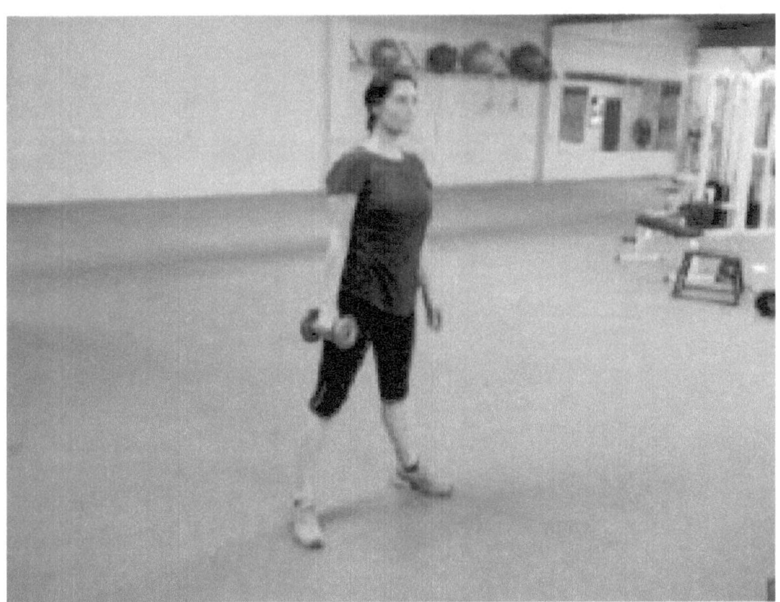

This exercise is thought to be complicated but essentially you are "jumping" the dumbbell up in one motion by utilizing every muscle in your body and burning tons of calories. Jump the dumbbell above your head, pushing through the dumbbell as you're squatting down. Return to the starting position and repeat.

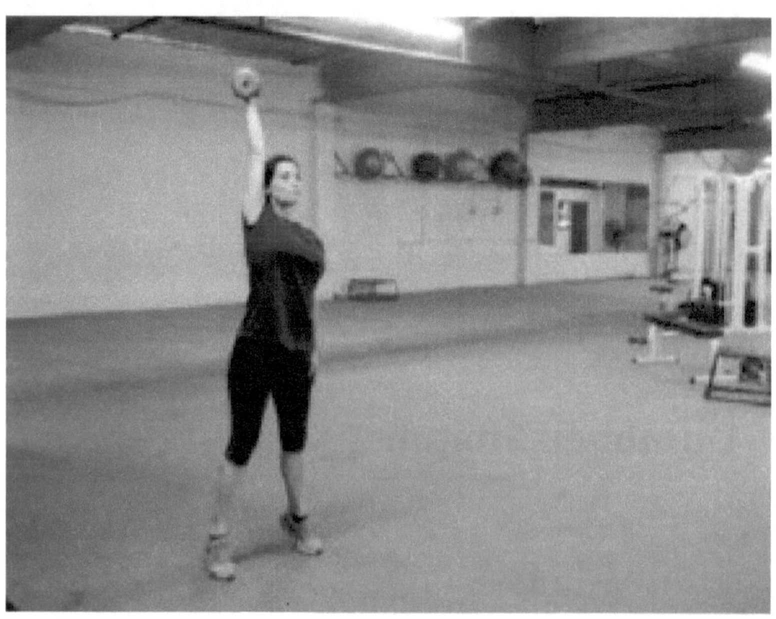

Walk-Outs

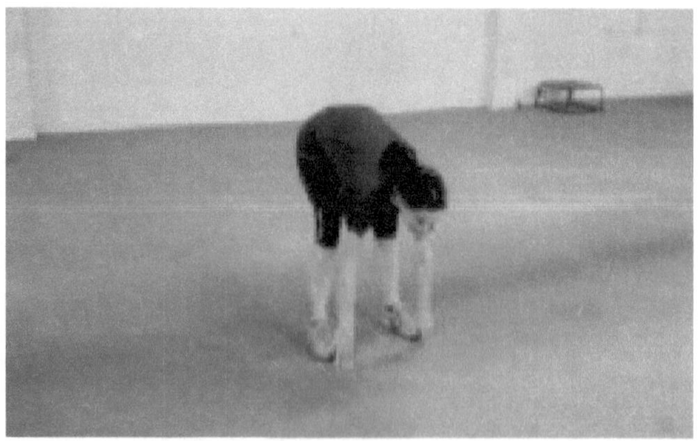

Start in a standing position. Bend your knees and walk your hands walk out onto the floor then slowly bring them back, as you see in the pictures. Make sure that every time you come back, you start back in the standing position.

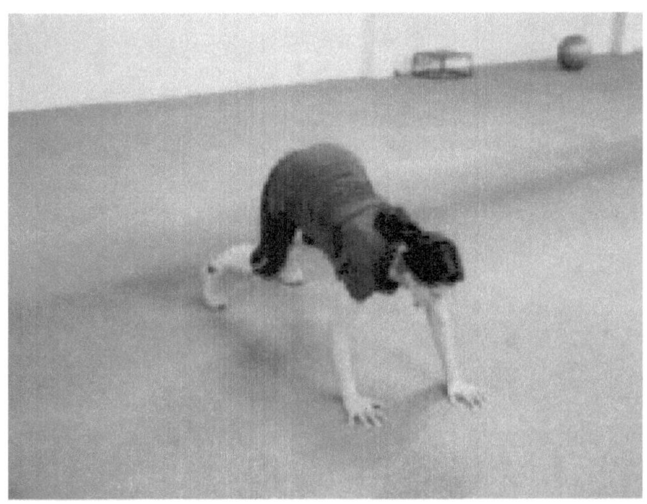

Windshield Wipers

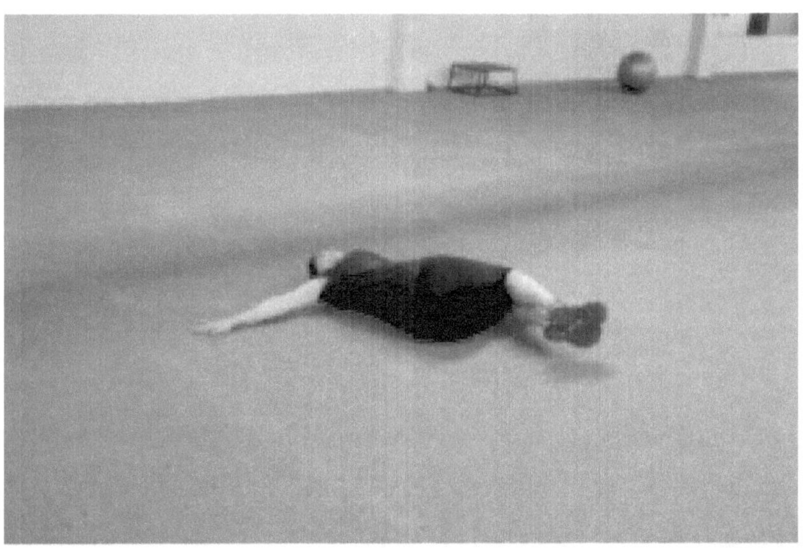

Lie on your back with your hips and knees bent at roughly a 90-degree angle. Keep your hands flat and out to your side. Now, move your hips from side to side while keeping your feet and knees together.

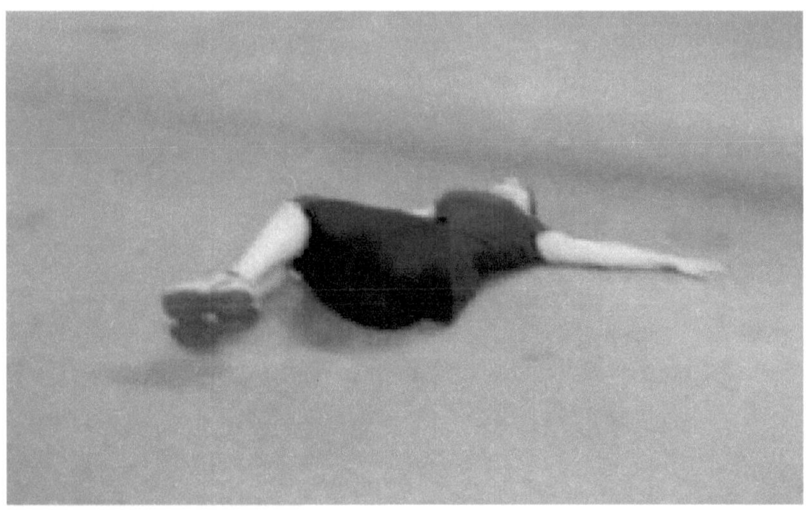

Floor Bridge

Lay flat on your back with your arms out to your side and your feet on the ground. Raise your hips toward the sky while squeezing your glutes. Bring your hips back to floor. Repeat the movement.

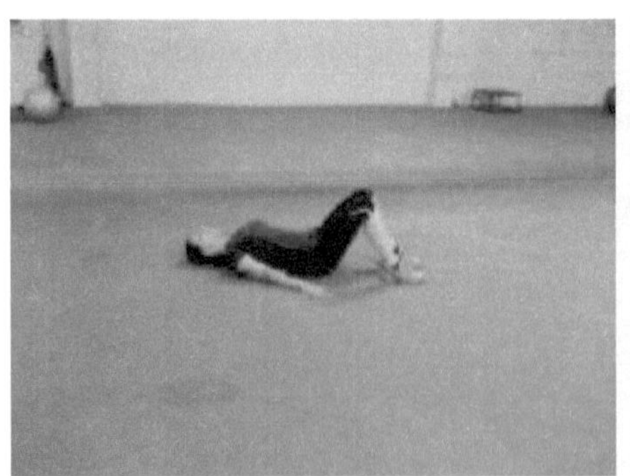

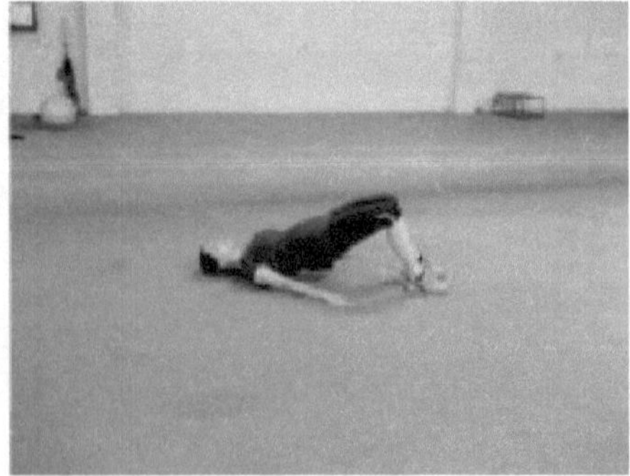

Push - Plate

To get in the starting position, place a weight plate in front of you. Crouch down and place both hands on the plate. Push the plate by driving the balls of your feet into the ground. Push for 20 to 30 yards and return to the starting point.

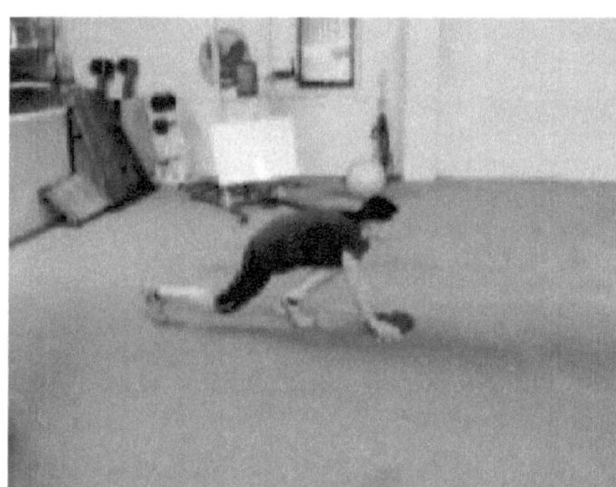 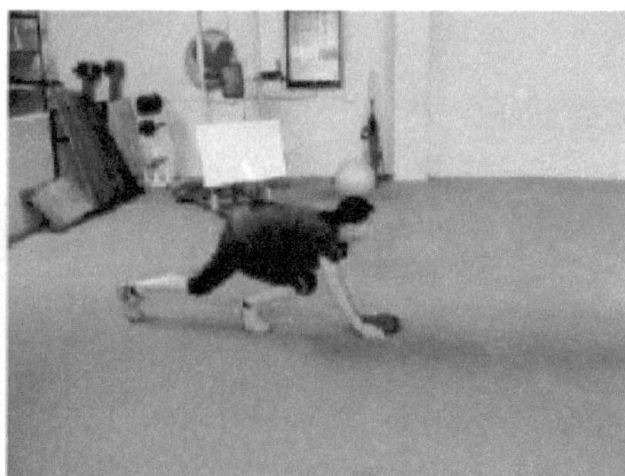

Reverse Crunch

Lay flat on your back with your legs raised, as seen in the pictures. Pull your knees toward your chest, keeping your feet off the ground. Return to the starting position. Repeat the movement.

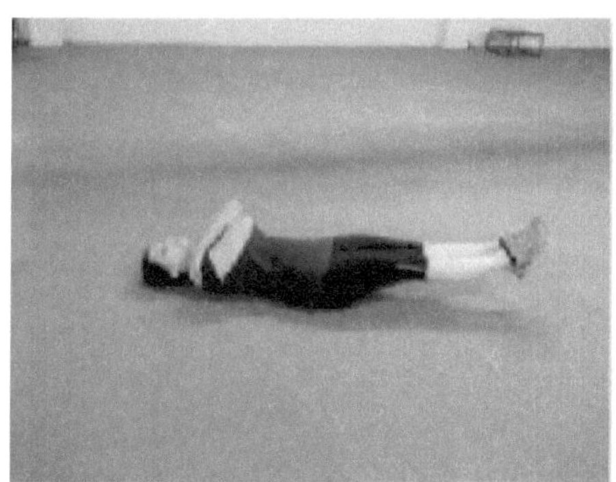 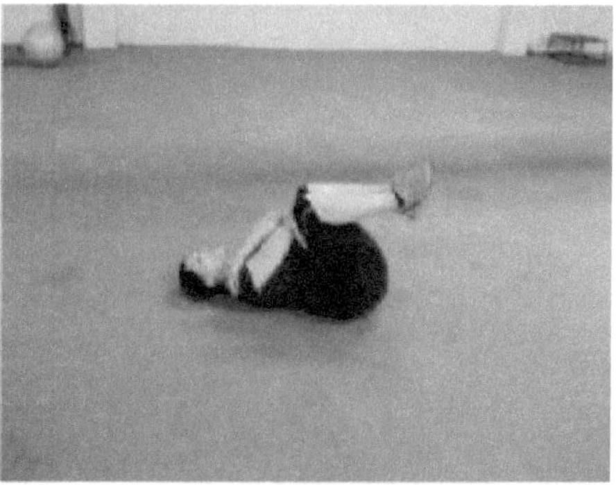

Workout Programs

Beginners

This section contains five different workout sequences for beginners. For each of the workouts:

1. Perform each exercise for 8 reps with a 30-second rest between exercises. Complete three circuits with no rest between the circuits.
2. Perform each exercise for 10 reps with no rest between exercises. Complete four circuits with a one-minute rest between circuits.
3. Perform each exercise for 12 reps. Complete as many circuits as you can in 10 minutes.
4. Group three exercises into one group, and three exercises in the other do 15 reps for one and 10 reps for the other. Complete four circuits with a 20-second rest between exercises and no rest between sets.
5. Perform each exercise for 20 reps with no rest between exercises. Complete four circuits. Rest for two minutes between circuits.

Note: For the Plank and Superman exercises, your initial goal is to hold the exercise for 30 seconds and build up to one minute. For cardio exercises, your initial goal is to complete 10 seconds of cardio and then build up to 30 seconds.

Workout #1	Workout #2
Squat	Dumbbell Squat Thrusts
Plank	Dumbbell Row
Jumping Jacks	(Bench) Dips
Push-Ups	Side Shuffle
Windmills	Windhsield Wipers
Lunges	High Pulls

Workout #3	Workout #4	Workout #5
Beginners Recline Pull	Step-Ups	Upright Row
Alt Splits Squats	Good Morning	Farmer's Walk
Floor Bridge	Barbell Front Suqat	Alternate Dumbbell Row
Dumbbell Snatch	Dumbbell Russian Twist	Run in Place
Dumbbell Chest Press	Dumbbell Shoulder Press	Criss Cross Jumping
Jacks Sprint Lateral	Squat Superman	

<u>Intermediate</u>

This section contains five different workout sequences for intermediates. For each of the workouts:

1. Perform each exercise for 15 reps. One circuit should last 15 minutes. Complete as many circuits as possible, with no rest between circuits, and keep track of how many circuits you complete.
2. Organize the exercises into groups of two, creating three sets of two exercises in each

group. Perform 30 reps for the first group, 20 reps for the second group, and 10 reps for the third group. Do as many rounds as you can in fifteen minutes.

3. Organize the exercises into three groups, with one group of three, one group of two, and the last group with one. For the group with three, perform each exercise for 45 seconds and do as many reps as you can during that time. For the group of two, perform each exercise for 30 seconds and do as many as you can in 30 seconds. For the last group, perform each exercise for 15 seconds and do as many as you can in that time. Complete three circuits with a one-minute rest between circuits.

4. Put the exercises into a group of five and do 15 reps for each exercise, with no rest between exercises. Go to the last exercise and perform 100 reps. Split the reps in sets of 25 if you can't perform all 100 at one time. Complete three rounds for each circuit, with a two-minute rest between circuits.

5. Perform 50 reps for two exercises, with a 30-second rest between those exercises and perform 25 reps for the remaining four exercises, with no rest between exercises. Complete three circuits with a one-minute rest between circuits.

Note: For Planks and the Superman, hold for one minute and build to two minutes. Perform the cardio exercises for

30 seconds and build to one minute.

Workout #1	Workout #2
DB Push Jerk	Sprint
Alternate Dumbbell Chest Press	Superman
Alt Rotational Dumbbell Row	Dumbbell Push Press
Rotational Plank	Reverse Lunge
Lunge	Pull Ups
Cross Overs	Barbell Deadlift

Workout #3	Workout #4	Workout #5
T-Bar Row	Recline Pulls	Lunge
High-Pulls	Dumbbell Swing	Rotational Deadlift
RDL's	One Legged Dumbbell Deadlift	Jumping JAcks
Side Plank	Diamond Push-Ups	Up-Downs
Dumbbell Rows	Step-Ups w/ Weights	Incline Push-Ups
Standing DB Shoulder Press	Waiter's Walk	Chin-Ups

Advanced

This section contains five advanced workout sequences. For each of the workouts:

1. Perform each exercise for 30 seconds and complete as many reps as possible in that time. Do not rest between exercises. Complete the circuit four times, rest for one minute after every circuit.
2. Perform 10 reps for each exercise for 25

minutes. Go through each circuit with no rest until 25 minutes have elapsed. Perform as many circuits as possible. Keep track of how many circuits you perform and track your improvement.

3. Perform alternating high reps (20) and low reps (8) for each exercise. If you're using bodyweight exercises, do 12 reps and repeat each circuit five times, with a thirty-second rest after the heavy exercises (low reps) and a one-minute rest between circuits. Have a barbell and dumbbell set up ahead of time to perform the circuits.

4. Perform five reps (find a weight for which you can't perform more than five reps and for which you can perform at least five reps) for all barbell and dumbbell exercises. For bodyweight exercises, do 30 reps per exercise and rest for 45 seconds between each circuit. Perform four circuits.

5. Perform each exercise for four minutes. There are six exercises per group. Break the time up for each exercise in preferably one-minute increments unless you can go for four minutes straight. Rest for 30 seconds between increments and for one minute between exercises.

Note: Hold the Planks and Supermans for two minutes then build to three minutes. Perform cardio for one minute and build to two minutes.

Workout #1	Workout #2
Snatch Dumbbell	Rotational Plank
Clap Push-Up	Walking DB Swings
Alt Split Squats	Turkish Get Up
Deadlift Dumbbell	Push Jerk
Barbell Squat	Barbell Hang Clean
Walkouts	Up-Downs

Workout #3	Workout #4	Workout #5
Bus Driver's	Crab Walks	Side Bear Crawl
Bulgarian Squats	Reverse Lunge	Plate - Push
Clean & Jerk	Lateral DB Swing	Box Jump
Good Mornings	Dips	DB Overhead Squat
Bear Crawls	Rotational Push Ups	Barbell Shovel
Dumbbell Russian Twists	Alt Split Squats	Waiters Walk

There you have it. You now know The Ultimate Women's Fat Loss System, the best fat-burning, muscle-building exercises on the planet. These exercises and routines can literally change your life and, along with the nutritional program, can lead you down a path of health and fitness for many years to come. You can now look forward to increased energy and productivity at work and around the house. In a sense, life has just got much easier. Yes, you will have to work your a** off to accomplish your goals, but because you have made the decision to start a resistance training program, other tasks and activities will become much easier.

`The confidence, and self-esteem that you will gain, not

only from the new body you have built, but from your discipline, consistency, and work ethic in shaping the body of your dreams, will be evident not only to yourself, but to everyone around you. Goals from other aspects of your life will seem attainable, and tasks that seemed insurmountable can now be conquered. There is literally nothing that can hold you back.

[1] Agricultural Marketing Service—National Organic Program [Online]. United States Department of Agriculture. Available at: http://www.ams.usda.gov/nop/ (verified 8 Dec 2008).

[2] http://organicecology.umn.edu

[3] Requirements chart written and updated by Jim Riddle on December 20, 2006.

[4] Source of stats: Whole Foods Market Organic Trend Tracker

[5] Winter, CK and SF Davis, 2006 "Organic Foods" Journal of Food Science

www.ingramcontent.com/pod-product-compliance
Lightning Source LLC
Chambersburg PA
CBHW031232250726
48655CB00005B/1925